Unshakable Awareness

Meditation in the Heart of Chaos

Other books by Richard L. Haight

The Warrior's Meditation
The Unbound Soul
Inspirience: Meditation Unbound
The Psychedelic Path

Unshakable Awareness

Richard L. Haight

Shinkaikan Body, Mind, Spirit LLC
www.richardlhaight.com

ISBN 978-1-7349658-1-0

Disclaimer:
1. Some names and identifying details have been changed to protect the privacy of individuals.
2. This book is not intended as a substitute for the medical or psychological advice of physicians or psychiatrists. The reader should regularly consult health practitioners in matters relating to his or her physical or mental/emotional health and particularly with respect to any symptoms that may require diagnosis or medical attention.

Published by Shinkaikan Body, Mind, Spirit LLC
www.richardlhaight.com

Table of Contents

Acknowledgments

Unshakable Awareness is dedicated to my martial arts instructor, Shizen Osaki (June 17, 1951 – July 27, 2020). He was a great mentor and a dear friend. I cannot thank him enough for all he has done to support my path and the Total Embodiment Method. If not for him, this book could not have been written. His spirit lives on through his children and his many students.

I would like to thank my students Barbara Becker, Linda LaTores, and Toni Hollenbeck for their early feedback on the manuscript and their suggesting a workbook be appended to the main text. They provided most of the questions that make up the workbook.

I would also like to thank my mentoring students for positively tackling the many challenges that this training offers and for their many questions, which have served to clarify the content of this book.

To my copy-editor, Hester Lee Furey, I extend my most sincere appreciation for the great work that she does and for her support of these teachings.

I thank my proofreading team, Barbara Becker, Linda LaTores, Toni Hollenbeck, and Rhoann Ponseti, for their quest to find every last error!

I thank the cover designer, Nathaniel Dasco, for the stunning design. He never ceases to amazing me.

I thank my wife, Teruko Haight, for her undying support of my awareness explorations.

Finally, I offer gratitude to the many supporters who financially contributed to help pay for the publishing of this book. Please know that I couldn't have done this without your support.

Below, I list each contributor by name:

John Roscoe
Linda LaTores
Leila Atbi
Rhoann Ponseti
Vinod Shakyaver
Ziad Masri
Toni Hollenbeck
Aleksandra Ivanov
Matthew Jones
Jean Jacques Rousseau
Harvey Newman
Colleen Scott
Thomas Kennedy
Jason Wu
Brian Darby
Ana Cinto
Clive Johnston
Wanda Aasen
Ryan J Pitts
Barbara Becker
Mark Lyon

From the depths of my heart, I thank you all!

Preface

As I type these words, billions of people are in self-isolation, unable to leave their homes, and many of them are also unable to work. Millions of people are sick with the corona virus (COVID-19), and thousands are dying miserably each day because we lack sufficient testing, hospital beds, and ventilators. The stock market is tanking, having lost almost half its value in only a few weeks, a decline far worse than the Great Depression of 1929 (during which it took three years for the market to lose half its value). The price of crude oil has dropped into the $20 per barrel range, prompting oil producers to clamor for a bailout because most of them can't survive at such low prices. Will these things rebound or not, nobody knows, for we are in a time of chaos.

For years "preppers" have been getting ready for an utter collapse of the modern system. Just a few months ago, almost no one took them seriously; now ordinary people are hoarding water, food, ammunition, and toilet paper. Even in the United States in cities where most citizens identify as liberal, such as New York and California, ammunition sales are outpacing stores' ability to stock their shelves.

Many of us are scared. We've never been in a situation like we are in now, but the fact is, whether we want to believe it or not, we are here, and we don't know what will come next. Time, a formerly rare commodity, has come to seem abundant for most of us as we remain at home in social isolation. Once we admit our condition, we can begin initiating positive action toward better health, inner strength, and awareness with the time that we have.

Not only do we have an abundance of time, we also have the lurking fear that our system may never recover, and that life as we have known it is gone. We're not sure what our future looks like.

Wishful thinking says that everything will return to normal in a few months. I understand how seductive such thinking can be, but it may not be as helpful as it seems at first glance, as it can lull us into inactivity and keep us in old, unhelpful patterns. Instead, we can use such moments to notice how we have been living in ways that are unhealthy, uninspiring, hollow of meaning, and unsupportive of our long-term well-being, by our own assessment.

While it is nice to hope for the best, we are wise to prepare for the worst. Maybe we don't have the money to purchase a gun, horde food, buy a fallout shelter, or whatever else that so many people are doing now. But we have another way to prepare. We can invest in the one thing that most people, including "preppers" tend to neglect: the fitness of our mind, body, and spirit. Of course, if you can establish secure access to shelter, water, and food, then you might consider doing so.

The truth is, even if you have prepared shelter, water, and food, if you have not conditioned your body, mind, and spirit to be powerfully capable under pressure, then you will not perform or live as well as you would otherwise. Consider a person lost in the forest. Most individuals who die in that circumstance do so because they panic and begin walking before calming themselves. They may walk for hours, possibly following someone's tracks, but ultimately end up exhausting themselves. They often die alone in fear. The sad part is that often the tracks they are following are their own, as they walk a large circle over the wilderness time and again, not realizing that they have been circling toward their primary arm over a span of miles.

If they weren't so physically and psychologically overwhelmed, they might have noticed more of their environment and made wiser choices that could have saved their lives. Because we are so insulated in the modern world, we often fail to recognize that the condition of our body, mind, and spirit is central to everything that we have ever experienced and everything that we will ever experience. Not only does the health of this triune being determine the base quality of our lives, it also determines the degree to which we are able to flow with pressure before we become overwhelmed.

This book is meant to help you tune up your mind, body, and spirit through ancient training methods of the Samurai and other traditions of the distant past. Through practicing these time-tested methods, not only will your physical health likely improve, so too will your mental clarity and emotional stability improve.

Through dedicated practice of the methods shown here, you will find you are able to tap into resources of calm clarity and capability under extreme pressure you had not realized were available for you. Your life will start to feel more interconnected with the people and the environment around you, which creates a certain motivating meaning. The quality of your daily life will improve.

This book is not meant to be a survival guide, but many of the principles within it may help to save lives in times of hardship, as it will serve to educate you on some very basic survival principles and ready your body, mind, and spirit for hard conditions.

Through these practices, your fitness and awareness will improve on all levels. The tendency to experience anxiety, panic, denial, depression, and feelings of meaninglessness will drastically reduce, and you will feel much more confident and powerful as a human being, more able to take up the challenges that we are likely to experience in a changing world.

Introduction

The methods taught in this book are born of ancient practices now often associated with religious rituals. In the ritualization of these practices, however, more often than not, something vital is lost: practicality.

To realize the true applications of these ancient practices, I have stripped away the ritualistic elements so you can focus on the essential principles. To help keep you invested in your training, I have also included a powerful progress assessment tool that will provide helpful feedback on your rate of improvement. The practices and the feedback system are readily accessible to people of any background or meditative experience-level, right at home.

But why would you trust me? What qualifies me to write this book? I've dedicated my life to Samurai training, meditation, and Japanese therapy arts, with the specific purpose of unifying body, mind, and spirit. In my pursuit, I spent 15 years in Japan studying with some of the most advanced teachers in the country, ultimately receiving master's licenses in four Samurai arts, as well as a therapy art called sotai-ho.

Based on the principles of ancient practices that I studied, I have formulated a new method of awareness training I call the "Total Embodiment Method (TEM)." TEM is inspired by the master Samurai who was vibrantly calm and aware, even amid the chaos of battlefield combat.

From the TEM curriculum, I wrote *The Warrior's Meditation*, which became a top-selling meditation book. *The Warrior's Meditation* is hailed as a revolutionary approach because it allows one to meditate through all activities of daily life, not only while in protected sedentary conditions.

The bottom line is that the Total Embodiment Method is meant to help you hold up to the pressures of life and death situations as well as the stresses and pressures of everyday life. Moreover, the practices taught will also help you to be calm and clear during long periods of isolation like those so many of us are experiencing now.

Through TEM training, your base physical, mental, and emotional fitness will improve, enabling you to deal with all aspects of life much more effectively than you could otherwise. Just as importantly, these methods will also help you to be at greater ease with the things that are not within your power to change.

Each tool that we will employ, including the progress assessment system, will serve to improve your physical, mental, and emotional health. As we will approach each of these ancient practices while meditated, we will be using some elements of the Warrior's Meditation, the foundational tool of the Total Embodiment Method, to help you get the most out of your experiences. Don't worry, the Warrior's Meditation is quite enjoyable, so boredom will likely not be a problem. Even children tend to find it easy and fun.

If you have already been practicing the Warrior's Meditation, know that you are going to receive a fresh take here that will expand your current understanding and meditative capabilities.

Psychology Today lists many scientifically verified benefits to meditation, benefits you will likely also gain from the exercises found in this book:

- Improved immune function, resulting in decreased cellular inflammation and pain
- Increased positive emotion through reduction of anxiety, depression, and stress
- Improved ability to introspect by providing a more holistic, grounded life perspective
- Improved social life from a boost in emotional intelligence and compassion with a reduction in feelings of insecurity
- Increased brain matter in areas related to paying attention, positive emotions, emotional regulation, and self-control
- Reduction in emotional reactivity
- Improved memory, creativity, and abstract thinking

These amazing benefits require a little cultivation to reach. Some become apparent quickly; others take time to manifest. To help you stay the course, in this book you receive a progress assessment tool to help you observe and reflect on your development as you practice. If you already employ another form of meditation, the principles shown here will blend well with what you are already practicing.

If you practice some of the religiously associated exercises, the stripped-down versions found in this book are designed to shine a light on the origins and mindsets of those who originally practiced the exercises, which should help you get the most out of your religious practice as well.

Not only will you practice meditative awareness, but you will intentionally make yourself progressively uncomfortable during your practice, so your awareness does not fail when you and loved ones are under stress, in pain, or in emergency situations.

While some of the exercises may at first glance seem extreme, know that they remain a normal and natural part of daily life for hunter-gatherers around the world. Furthermore, in some parts of the world, religious or ritualized forms of these methods are still common.

Recognize that our bodies evolved with these practices, and if done reasonably, they help our bodies to be vibrantly aware and healthy. Acknowledging the natural benefits of the exercises taught here helps us to have the right attitude toward them, so that we don't start feeding resistive narratives that may prevent us from gaining maximal benefit.

By strengthening our bodies, minds, and immune systems we develop a trusting relationship with the body that only comes from experiencing real challenges. Much in the way that we become stronger through the artificially induced stresses of weightlifting, we experience the deliberate discomfort of these exercises to reap the benefits.

Don't get me wrong; comfort has its time and place, but too much of it makes us weak on all levels. Just as we require an appropriate amount of comfort to sleep and digest well, for example, so too do our bodies, minds, and spirits need an optimal amount of discomfort to be fit.

The exercises are simple and safe, if practiced reasonably. I also provide methods that help you approach the practices through a graduated process, so you will not experience them as overwhelming or off-putting. The practices are easy; they can be performed right in your home. Furthermore, they are designed to blend with your daily life.

We all know how easily we can conjure excuses not to do healthy things that we should be doing. I know that my mind, if allowed, will try to avoid the training by coming up with rationalizations or by simply forgetting. To nullify that possibility, I designed all practices to be slight modifications to things that normal people must do every day. Since you need to perform these tasks anyway, it becomes difficult not to incorporate the training without knowing through and through that you are ducking out.

Initially, it is quite natural that one might desire to avoid challenging exercises, but as you practice them more and more, the immediate and longer-term benefits become quite clear. In the short term, how comparatively good you feel right after completing an exercise will certainly get your attention. From there, you can observe that you have more energy, think more clearly, are calmer, and get a lot more done during your day than you do when you skip these practices.

The benefits will keep you moving forward despite any momentary discomfort, and in so doing, you will realize you are capable of facing hardship and moving through it, which frees your mind and greatly empowers you in daily life.

Through these TEM practices you will establish a healthy, trusting body/mind relationship. Once a sufficient inner trust is established, you will see that your body has become your ally, no longer resisting your wise but sometimes challenging aims.

Through these practices, you will come to feel much more aware, positive, and confident during your daily life—incredibly important results. But there are some unexpected side-effects that I should mention:

You may experience moments of perfect blissful clarity or have spontaneous insights and solutions to problems that had previously seemed unsolvable.

You may also find that long-held, unresolved mental/emotional baggage and traumas begin to fade away.

Most certainly, you will feel much more present during daily life, possibly becoming aware of the pulse throughout your entire body.

You'll also become more aware of your environment. For example, some people report that they can feel when people are staring at them from behind or when they are nearing an unseen danger.

As your nervous system and mind tone sufficiently, you will likely experience heightened levels of intimacy and sexual pleasure, and you may experience periods of profound synchronicity, as if you were living in "The Zone."

Some individuals experience visionary states as a result of these practices. And many people report experiencing a feeling of transcendent oneness with all of life, which probably explains why variations of these practices have been incorporated into so many religions around the world.

As you begin your practice you may find yourself cursing my name, but I am confident that once you begin to see the benefits, you'll have nothing but good things to say. In either case, keep moving forward!

Finally, for individuals who have certain health conditions, I provide alternative practices that allow work toward greater health in smaller steps. Individuals who have severe heart conditions will want to consult their doctors prior to experiencing this training method.

Let's begin our practice!

How to Use This Book

This book is designed as a training manual, which means you will get a quite different understanding of the methods and mindsets offered here by enacting the practices than you will from simply reading. Absent the daily training that this book endorses, I suspect the book will not be very satisfying, because the inspiration and transformational value doesn't come from the reading so much as from the doing.

One strategy is to read the book straight through to get an overview of the training method and then read as you experience the training. The other strategy is read and practice as you go. In either case, documenting your progress in the workbook will greatly aid your training. Filling out the workbook as you proceed will not only help you to better see the key points of this training method, but also to more clearly perceive the invisible forces that might have blocked your awareness. You can find the Step-by-Step Workbook at the end of the book. If you would prefer to download and print it out, you can do so at the following URL:

https://richardlhaight.com/uaworkbook/

With daily application, you will soon begin to notice profoundly beneficial changes in your energy, attitude, thinking, feeling, commitment, and ability to follow through on your aims each day. Don't be surprised if your overall health starts to change for the better. Most importantly, your awareness will vastly expand.

Finally, remember that the training methods here are meant to be experienced at the pace of each individual. There is no point in rushing through the training as quickly as possible. Instead, move through at a pace that is challenging but not totally overwhelming. That said, persistence is the key to any life transformation, so be sure to show up for yourself and the training every day without fail.

With you in training,
Richard L. Haight

P.S. With this book, I am offering you a 30-day trial of my daily online guided meditation service, which means I will personally walk you through the steps of the Warrior's Meditation each day. You will find the link at the end of the book. Thousands of people are doing it every day!

Part 1

Mind-Body Restructuring

TEM training is designed to affect our bodies and minds in highly integrated ways that will, with practice, allow you to completely embody awareness or meditation in your daily life. People tend to think of meditation and awareness as a purely mental exercise. So long as we hold that view of meditation, the benefits that we could gain from the practice are greatly limited.

The truth is that most of us have highly embodied physical, mental, and emotional ruts that run much deeper than mere thought. To address these deeper issues requires training the body and the mind with a certain degree of disciplined behavior and self-study.

Through TEM training, we will address all three areas of stuckness: physical, mental, and emotional. To address these areas with success, it will be helpful for you to understand which systems of the body will change through the training and how those changes affect body, mind, and emotions.

The study of the mind-body restructuring will be integral in keeping you on the path, for you will quickly recognize the sometimes-counterintuitive signs of progress. If you can see the signs as they arise, even if you are uncomfortable, you will feel encouraged to continue with the training. All lasting progress will require persistent practice. Knowing how the mind and body restructure through this training will prove critical.

In Part I, you will learn about how your brain structures pathways in its process of learning and adapting to the moment and how you can intentionally restructure those neural pathways to optimize awareness in daily life. You will also learn about the bodily changes that occur at nervous system, cellular, and vascular levels as you progress through the training regimen. Those changes will provide you with more energy and resilience under pressure, so you can remain aware even when you feel uncomfortable.

Chapter 1

Neuroplasticity

Most people unconsciously assume that the way they think and feel now is how they will always think and feel, that the habits and addictions that may plague us will be with us for the rest of our lives. As people age, they tend to give up on their ability to learn and change, an attitude that is summed up by the idea of being "set in your ways."

In fact, no one is actually set in their ways, but that attitude can create the illusion of being stuck. Until very recently the scientific community tended to assume that the brain did not change much once an individual reached maturity. Over the years, however, a number of people with brain damage recovered in ways that made no sense if the brain were not capable of adapting. Research upon such individuals revealed that the brain is constantly rebuilding itself, dismantling unused neuropathways and building new ones to help the individual adapt to their changing environment all through the life of the individual.

With the undeniable observation that the brain is constantly changing, the attitude of being "set" in any way no longer makes much sense. Yes, many people do indeed seem set in their ways, which really means stuck in habits, but part of the reason they are stuck is the false assumption that being stuck is natural or inevitable because the brain cannot change. If you believe you are stuck and there is nothing that can be done about it, and then do not put in the necessary effort to break out of the habit, your belief is self-fulfilling. It is still incorrect, though.

To help you see beyond the limits of being "set," let's take a look at the neural network, known as the brain, to get a greater understanding of its incredible flexibility, known as neuroplasticity, and how we can begin to hack into this biological process to improve the quality of our lives.

Researchers at the Stanford University School of Medicine, using a state-of-the-art imaging system to scan brain-tissue, have revealed that the average human brain contains about 200 billion nerve cells, called neurons. Neurons link to other neurons via connection points called synapses; these points relay electrical impulses from one neuron to another.

We might imagine that a single neuron would connect to just one or a few other neurons, much like the wiring in a circuit board, but the reality is far more incredible. As it turns out, a single neuron may have tens of thousands of synaptic contacts with other neurons.

Considering the unbelievable interconnectivity of neurons, we might assume that each neuron is quite large, but we'd be wrong. Even with all the vast interconnectivity of neurons, individually they measure less than a thousandth of a millimeter in diameter.

If you've ever turned over a piece of wood or bark in a forest you may notice a complex of white tissue growing at the former connection points between the wood and the soil. That white material is called mycelium, which is the root system of fungi. Surprisingly, our brains' neurological matrix operates similarly to fungal mycelium, which also transmits signals through components like the synapse that are astoundingly small. The matrix is so complex and tightly knit that it is quite difficult to conceptualize the complexity of the "circuitry" that makes up our feeling, thinking, and motivational systems.

Astoundingly, a single neuron, even with its incredibly tiny measurement in physical space, contains phenomenal memory storage and processing capabilities. Stephen Smith, PhD, is a professor of molecular and cellular physiology who, with Kristina Micheva, PhD, invented Array tomography, an imaging method that allows us to see the true complexity of the brain. According to Smith, "One synapse, by itself, is more like a microprocessor—with both memory-storage and information-processing elements—than a mere on/off switch. In fact, one synapse may contain on the order of 1,000 molecular-scale switches. Now imagine your brain has 200 billion such mini processors working together" ("Stunning Details of Brain Connections Revealed").

Looking more closely at the memory held in neurons, we discover that each neuron is influenced by all the connected neurons and their memory associations. Each neuron potentially connects to tens of thousands of associations, which means the brain holds an ocean of memory, the vast majority of which is unconscious.

The truly fascinating aspect of this massive memory-hoard is that when the brain changes, memories and associations shift with it. This concept may seem extremely counterintuitive at first, until you learn that every time you access a memory, you are changing it. It turns out that as you access memory, aspects of your current circumstances get written into the memory, influencing it in unconscious ways. Because of the way memory is rewritten, many adults have false memories of their young childhood, based on stories that they were told by family members. A child may remember having an experience that they never actually had because they heard the story when they were young. The false memory, as vivid as it might seem, is the product of imagination.

Given the ever-changing nature of the brain and memory, we can begin to see how it is possible that our very sense of self can change in empowering or disempowering ways. Because most people's sense of self is driven by memory, as the brain changes, which it does every moment, memory changes subtly, as does the sense of self. Even if we are unaware of the change, it is happening.

Once we recognize that the brain constantly changes, we no longer need to be imprisoned by the belief that we are "set" in our ways, unless we want to continue being stuck. To enrich our lives, we are wise to consciously take advantage of the brain's ability to constantly remodel itself through the mechanism known as neuroplasticity.

We now know that whatever we pay attention to or practice during our waking hours gets reinforced in the brain when we sleep. During sleep, resources are removed from pathways that are not being used and allocated to the pathways that were stimulated during the day. Realizing how the brain changes, we can begin to consciously stimulate what we wish to reinforce in the brain.

If you are not practicing mindfulness in productive ways daily and if you are not getting sufficient sleep, then your process of life enrichment will be slowed. Assuming you practice and sleep reasonably well, you will make notable progress. Even a few minutes of conscious meditation practice every day helps. From my own experience and feedback from students, it is clear that even with disturbed sleep, the beneficial changes are accessible, but simply unfold at a slower pace.

The degree to which you engage with your meditative practice determines the degree to which the brain responds. If you take your training seriously and make it a priority in your life, you will likely reap notable benefits even in the short term. That said, the real transformation is found in the long game.

The reality we must face is that the brain is habituated to react to stimulus in certain disharmonious ways, ways that are counter to awareness, ways that create the effect of self-absorption. Realizing that we have counterproductive emotional and perspective-related habits, we can begin to make changes via the principle of neuroplasticity. The only question is whether you choose to take advantage of the opportunity to rewrite your brain each day.

Again, if you are elderly, you might worry that you have less potential to benefit from neuroplasticity than children, but do not let that concern stop you from taking positive action. Research is showing that with a healthy lifestyle and persistence over time, even seniors can promote productive brain change. Just keep moving forward each day toward greater awareness, and you will be far better off than you would be if you fell into complacency.

One of the main barriers you might encounter as you challenge existing brain patterns with new perspectives and practices is that awkward feelings might arise. Feeling awkward is unpleasant, to be sure, so it is understandable that we might want to avoid that experience. Avoiding awkwardness, however, often leads us away from progress, for awkwardness is a necessary part of learning.

To get an idea of what I mean, consider the difference in your ability to write or throw a ball with your dominant arm, compared to your other arm. Most of us are so accustomed to throwing a ball or writing with the same arm that we never use our non-dominant arm for those activities, resulting in complete ineptitude with the secondary limb and sometimes observable muscular imbalance between the two sides of the body. We have become addicted to the feeling of confidence that we get when we use our primary arm.

Actually, it's not only your secondary arm that is underdeveloped and dysfunctional, but also the neural pathways of the brain that pertain to that arm's functionality. Your brain is unfamiliar with writing or throwing a ball using the secondary arm because it lacks the stimulation that would allow it to familiarize a set of neural pathways related to those activities.

In the same way that throwing a ball or writing with your non-dominant hand may be awkward, many other important neural pathways may be underdeveloped that relate to awareness and the body-mind relationship. Through the training offered in this book, we will address those awkward areas so that new awareness, balance, and a healthier, more connected body-mind relationship can emerge.

The famous Japanese martial arts master, Takeda Sokaku, headmaster of Daito-ryu Aikijujutsu (the form of jujutsu that I study and teach), was able to use his sword equally well with either hand, something he trained himself to do. Traditionally speaking, one must draw and hold the sword with right hand dominant. Takeda Sensei felt that having an imbalanced ability was a weakness, so he made extra effort to balance his training. He had a distinct advantage over anyone who was trained to be right hand dependent.

As a result of his training, his swordsmanship became extremely flexible as did his mind and awareness. He could also use the short sword as well as he could the long sword, and two swords as well as one sword. Many of his students would recount how he was always training himself to do everything with his non-dominant hand, attempting to match the abilities of his primary hand. You would be wise to take a similar approach to your training, so you are constantly challenging your weaknesses in creative ways.

Although Takeda Sensei certainly did not know about neuroplasticity, he developed incredible abilities and became known as one of Japan's greatest martial artists. After hearing of his training methods, I began using my non-dominant hand more often with tasks that I had previously only executed with my right hand. For example, I began to eat using chopsticks in my left hand instead of my right. It took a few weeks to train my brain to use chopsticks left-handed, but before long, Japanese people were complimenting me on how well I used chopsticks. They were shocked when I told them that I was not left-handed, and they usually admitted that they could not use chopsticks with their secondary hand. For fun, I would grab another pair of chopsticks with my right hand and eat with both hands like a crab.

To get an idea of how your brain pattern allows your bodily functionality, try the following exercise:

Pick up a pen and write your name with your primary hand and notice how easy and natural it feels. Next, change the pen over to your other hand and try writing your name with it. Observe how awkward it feels. Notice also how hard you must concentrate compared to using your primary hand. The effort you feel is not so much located in the muscles of your arm but within your brain, as it seeks to make neurological connections to allow the movement. Once those connections are sufficiently developed, writing with your non-dominant hand will no longer feel awkward.

Writing is a relatively difficult challenge for our non-dominant hand to accomplish, so it serves as an obvious way to demonstrate your brain's current limitation and how it feels as it links new neural pathways. As we go through the exercises in this book, keep in mind that when your brain is building neural pathways it feels awkward and uncomfortable. What this means is that as soon as any exercise feels easy and comfortable, to keep improving, you need to make it a little more challenging, so as to stimulate further neurological development.

Powerful benefits emerge when we approach training in this neurologically conscious way. The first is that our training will be less ego driven because we will know without a doubt that working only on what makes us look good or feel comfortable does not sufficiently challenge us. As we develop abilities and refine them through the awkward, uncomfortable feelings that come of learning to do anything that is challenging, the brain will also learn that the effort and discomfort needed to improve are worth the investment.

Most importantly, the brain will learn that it can face hardships and moving through them to improve, which changes your entire outlook on life. Whatever life brings becomes your means of refinement on so many levels: physical, mental, and emotional/spiritual. Every moment is an opportunity!

Chapter 2

Vagal Nerve Stimulation

Now that we have an understanding of how the brain changes and how we can consciously guide those changes for self-improvement, it's time to get a sense of how the nervous system and body will change as a result of the TEM training exercises that we explore in the upcoming chapters.

The first and most obvious change will come through stimulation of the vagal nerve, which is one of nine cranial nerves. The vagal nerve manages a vast array of vital functions by conveying motor and sensory impulses to the organs. The vagal nerve connects your brainstem to your visceral organs, through which it controls the parasympathetic nervous system, and helps to counteract the fight-flight-freeze adrenal responses of the sympathetic nervous system, such as stress, anxiety, depression, and panic.

These sympathetic responses cause much of the mental, emotional, and physical pain that many of us experience each day. Aside from priming the mind and emotions for hyper-reactivity and bodily inflammation, fight-flight-freeze responses also cause many of the blunders that we tend to make when under pressure.

Fortunately, we have many ways to stimulate the vagal nerve so as to shift out of the stressful fight-or-flight mode and into the rest-and-digest mode of the parasympathetic nervous system. Rest-and-digest is the mode that our bodies would be in 90% of the time if we lived as hunter-gatherers, which is the way our bodies evolved to live.

So that you may recognize when your training is stimulating the vagal nerve and shifting your nervous system, let's learn a little about the science of vagal stimulation.

Research has shown many health benefits to vagal stimulation, which

- Prevents inflammation by helping to regulate proper immune response
- Improves communication between the gut and the brain to provide a more precise intuition
- Improves memory by triggering norepinephrine to be released into the amygdala, which consolidates memories
- Improves heartbeat regulation through electrical impulses to muscle tissue in the right atrium
- Initiates the body's relaxation response through the release of acetylcholine, prolactin, vasopressin, and oxytocin
- Reduces or prevents symptoms of rheumatoid arthritis, hemorrhagic shock, and other serious inflammatory diseases formerly thought to be incurable.

As you can see, vagal nerve stimulation has profound impacts on the body and mind, so practicing various forms of vagal stimulation will contribute significantly to achieving a higher quality of life and becoming a more aware individual.

In subsequent chapters we will experiment with various methods, all of which are helpful in toning the vagal nerve to stimulate the aforementioned scientifically verified benefits. To get some idea of how powerful vagal nerve stimulation can be, try the following exercise:

Note: The vagal breathing method taught here is extremely powerful and can easily lead to instant blood pressure drops that could cause a fainting spell. Aside from the danger of a fall, there are no other negative effects of this method. Note also, my reference to "vagal breathing" should not be associated with other traditions that may use the same term applied to a slightly different practice.

1. Sit down to keep you safe in the event that you faint.
2. Take in a full breath and hold it while tensing your entire body. Be sure to tense the face as well. Hold the tension along with the breath.
3. Although it may seem as if your lungs are full, that is not actually the case. Without exhaling the current air in your lungs, inhale again to fully top off your lungs.
4. Hold the air and physical tension for as long as you can.
5. When you can no longer hold your breath, exhale slowly and relax the body. Allow your body to breathe naturally.

Notice how much calmer and more relaxed you feel after taking just one vagal breath. If you had measured your blood pressure and heart rate before and after this one breath, you would see a notable change. Through that one full breath, held for a short time, you stimulated the vagal nerve which communicates with the rest of your body and brings it into a relaxed, yet aware state.

You would be wise to practice vagal breathing a little each day as you have time. Vagal stimulation is extremely powerful and healthy. Due to its whole-body effect on health and awareness, all TEM practices include an element of vagal stimulation.

The changes in feeling and in the pulse, as well as many more you may not have noticed occur every time you stimulate the vagal nerve. If you can remember to stimulate the vagal nerve consciously every day, you have already enhanced the fundamental quality of your life in an obvious way.

Although I do not mention vagal breathing as I explain the other activities of this book, you can combine the method you just learned with the other activities that we are going to explore in upcoming chapters as you like. Doing so, you may be surprised at how quickly it transforms your life.

Chapter 3

Other Bodily Changes

Along with the benefits of consciously guiding neuroplasticity, toning of the vagal nerve, and the subsequent improvements in heart-rate variation that vagal stimulation brings, we have recourse to several other scientifically verified healthy changes that occur in the body as a result of TEM training. In this chapter, we are going to learn about those changes and how they will serve to benefit our lives on physical, mental, and emotional levels.

Circulatory System

Several practices that we incorporate into our meditative training strengthen the circulatory system by toning the muscles within the walls of blood vessels: the arteries, arterioles, veins, and venules.

This toning allows the blood vessels to optimally adjust their diameter to maintain appropriate blood pressure and blood flow even when the body is under severe pressure. Toning the muscles of the vascular system allows them to dilate more effectively to accommodate required changes in blood volume according to the circumstances of the body.

The result of well-toned circulatory muscles is a body that is much more capable of handling pressure of all sorts and maintaining its strength and endurance. The question you may be asking yourself is, "How does the muscular strength of my blood vessels affect my awareness?"

It's an important question. Think back to moments in your life of feeling sickly, weak, exhausted, or overwhelmed. During those times, in all likelihood, your emotional state and thinking were also out of sorts, which means you were not tuned into awareness. As we seek to remain aware and meditated even under pressures and stressors that would cause other people to lose control of their minds, having a strong circulatory system is required.

This teaching is not new. In fact, legend has it that the reason that monks began to practice Shaolin Kung-fu is because they had grown so feeble from sedentary meditation that they would constantly fall asleep. Bodhidharma, the monk who is credited for bringing Chan Buddhism to China, is said to have devised training methods to help strengthen monks so they would no longer fall asleep during their practice.

The legend says that Bodhidharma recommended martial art and breath training as a means of improving their meditation practice. These practices combined with the local martial arts and became what we now know of as Shaolin Kung-fu.

While the Kung-fu of today is likely quite changed from the way it was practiced back then, nonetheless, the point remains that physical conditioning is important to our health on all levels. If you are not interested in kung fu, do not worry, for we will not be learning martial arts techniques in this book. We have other means of developing the body. But before we get to those methods, let's learn a bit about the types of changes that will benefit us.

Cellular Changes

Mitochondria are organelles within cells that have their own distinct genetic code. Mitochondria are not human cells, but apparently the remnants of a biological symbiosis that occurred millions of years ago in multicellular organisms, wherein a bacterium entered a cell and performed the beneficial duty of providing many metabolic tasks for the cell, most notably producing energy.

If indeed the theory of symbiosis between bacteria and multicellular organisms holds true, the relationship appears to have worked tremendously well for all involved. In any case, that bacterium became a permanent part of animal life - a lasting partnership, in which the mitochondria provide for the energy needs of cells, freeing them up to focus on other vital activities. Your bodily heat and energy primarily come from the workings of those little mitochondria in your cells—gratitude is in order!

Whether you know it or not, the mitochondria are doing their job. You might wonder why we bother to learn about them. They are significant to our studies here because through the application of certain exercises, you can increase the mitochondrial count of your cells, thus protecting and potentially upgrading your body's vital energy. Studies have shown that on average mitochondrial function and count decrease as bodies age. A 40-year-old person has but a fraction of the cellular energy output that they had when they were born.

When cellular mitochondria become weak and/or numerically insufficient to fuel cellular functions, the body responds less efficiently to stress and suffers more from the pressures of life. On mental and emotional levels, if our bodies are weak, we will have less mental acuity, and we will experience more anxiety, more depression, and more negative emotion than we would otherwise (Pizzorno). Protect your mitochondria, for healthy abundant mitochondria positively affect your overall health (Bratic and Larsson).

There are still many questions about mitochondria and how they relate to aging and health that remain to be answered. But what we have seen is that the condition of mitochondria strongly correlates with the overall condition of our health and our aging process. Ridding the body of unhealthy cells, cells that have weak mitochondria or are otherwise compromised, while protecting healthy cells, appears to be essential to good health. Another key to vibrant health seems to be promoting the development of more mitochondria.

In summary, the Total Embodiment Method synergizes a number of powerful ancient practices that tune up your brain and strengthen the body at cellular levels as well as the immune, circulatory, and nervous systems, all of which have direct benefits to body, mind, and emotional health.

Let's do this!

Part II

Vagal Toning

Many ancient cultures believed that words and names had a divine spirit with creative power. In fact, more than most any other spiritual concept, the idea that words have supernatural power can be found in almost every ancient society around the world.

For example, devotees of ancient Christianity adhered to the belief that the Word of God, commonly referred to as the Logos in Greek, was imbued with divine creative power from which the universe sprang into being. The Hindus of India believe that Mantra, spiritual utterances or sounds derived from Sanskrit, had spiritual and or psychological powers and could influence human lives in supernatural ways.

This concept also appears in ancient Japanese culture in the term *kotodama*. The Japanese word *kotodama* is made up of the Chinese character *koto* (言), which translates as "sound," "word," or "language," and the Chinese character *dama* (霊), which can be translated as "soul," "spirit," "divine," or "sacred." The basic idea is that sound, words, and language have a spiritual nature, in that they are alive and filled with creative power which influences our physical, mental, emotional states, and even our environment. The idea that language has divine power may seem absurd to modern people, but when viewed from the perspective of the ancients, who were far more in touch with nature than we are and who lacked a scientific framework to describe their perceptions, it makes sense.

We will begin Part II by exploring some foundational sounds from the perspective of ancient people, so that we can begin to understand why the belief that language and sound are sacred can be found in every ancient culture around the globe. Once you understand that perspective, you will be ready to receive the benefits of a principled, secular sound practice. With a functional view of language and sound as it pertains to awareness, we will explore the dimensionality of sound as we produce it with our own bodies. This practice serves to significantly enhance our receptivity to subsequent practices and boost our awareness as a whole.

Finally, with the newly developed awareness of the nature of sound and enhanced bodily awareness of sound, you will learn how to feel which sounds provide the greatest therapeutic value for your body at any given time. The sensitivity and awareness developed through the practices found in Part II will serve as a foundation for all subsequent exercises.

Chapter 4

Primary Sounds

Ancient people recognized that human beings are infinitely more capable of "creating" and modifying our environment than are other animals. From the perspective of first peoples, who lived close to the earth, every creature is a relative. From the idea that we are relatives to other creatures, it is only natural to wonder why humans have so much more power to influence our environment than other animals.

Seeing that their power was not found in tooth and claw, as it is for most other creatures, early humans realized their strength lay in thought. They also realized that thought is structured by language, a structure that comes from the ancestors and transcends the individual.

Language, from their perspective, was a divine inspiration that traces back to the beginnings of humanity. They realized that if an individual wants to affect change in the world, he or she must first be able to imagine the desired change by seeing the future and then mentally articulating the path to that future.

If the plan requires the help of others, then it must be spoken to them. If the words are clear, inspiring, and in alignment with the needs or desires of the people, they will support the plan with the power of their language and physical effort.

Surely, we can see that we humans are genetic relatives to all other creatures, and we have an incredible creative power that allows us to modify our environment (for good or for ill) well beyond that of other creatures. The power of words helped us to survive in a dangerous world without claw, fang, or fur—a miraculous accomplishment. Considering that fact, it is easy to see why the word would be considered vitally important to the ancients—sacred even.

The sacredness of language, from the ancient's perspective, has its origin in raw sound vibration. Let's look at the very foundation of language, the vowel sounds. Vowel sounds A, I, U, E, O provide the foundational vibrations that give rise to language systems around the world, which are then modified by consonants, pauses, glottal stops, et cetera.

Vowel sounds are made with the mouth and throat unblocked throughout the sound. The sound of consonants, by contrast, entail sound being stopped or cut by the teeth, tongue, lips, or constriction of the vocal cords. To get a sense of what I mean by the vibrations of vowel sounds, you will need to vocalize the sounds with your whole body as one might do during a chant. Let's try chanting the "Ah" sound first while feeling the resulting vibration in the body. Make the sound loudly and from as low a place in your body as possible. When you make the "Ah" sound properly, you will notice that the vibrations seem to travel down the body.

Now let's compare a typical consonant sound like K. When you try to chant the K, which would be "KEH," the K part of the sound is temporary, at the very beginning of the chant, and cannot be maintained more than an instant. K quickly falls away leaving the "Eh" sound.

From experience, we can see that the K sound is definite, in that there is no way to sustain that sound, whereas the "Eh" sound can continue for an entire breath, which means that it is indefinite. That which is definite is mundane and that which is indefinite is transcendent.

Because the "Eh" sound continues and can mix with any sound and can take any position when making more complex sounds, it could be considered transcendent or sacred. By this measure, K and other sounds that cannot be sustained are considered mundane or ordinary sounds. To avoid unnecessary mysticism in our training, we will define all transcendent sounds as primary sounds and keep to that definition as your training moves forward.

By the definitions set out in the previous paragraph, we can see why the vowel sounds A, I, U, E, and O can be thought of as transcendent (primary) and why most consonants would be considered mundane (secondary) sounds. There are a few consonant sounds that fit the description of primary sounds. Note that the N and M sounds, which are consonants in English, like A, I, U, E, and O, create sustainable vibrations when chanted regardless of where they show up in a word.

Try it and see for yourself. They are not considered to be vowels in English because they are produced with a closed element (the lips for M and the tongue against the teeth for the N sound.) For our purposes, because M and N sounds are sustainable, they too are treated as primary sounds.

What about the "sometimes Y," you might wonder. Y is not a primary sound because when it behaves as a vowel in English, for example, in the word Hymn, the Y is vocalized as the vowel I, which produces a sustainable vibration. Thus, "Hymn" is actually pronounced "Him." When Y takes on its own sound, for example in "yellow," the Y sound is unsustainable, so it has the properties of a consonant.

You might wonder why knowing the difference between primary and secondary sounds matters to individuals who do not believe in the sacred. Primary sounds, when their vibrations are extended, as happens when chanting, stimulate the vagal nerve, which in turn improves physical, mental, and emotional health as we discussed in Chapter 2.

You will gain the benefits of primary sound vocalization regardless of beliefs. It turns out that chanting is an ancient survival technique. Sustaining vibrant health was vital to survival when humans were not so insulated from the elements, so the ancients took advantage of these sounds.

As we discussed earlier, primary sounds serve two amazing functions. They form the basis of language, which is the foundation of our thinking and our remarkable adaptive powers. Primary sound vibrations also benefit our health on physical, mental, and emotional levels. Just as primary sounds benefitted the lives of the ancients, so too can they benefit our lives if we utilize them.

To get some experience with these sounds, try mixing and matching the sounds "Ah," "Ee," "Ew," "Eh," "Oh," "Mmm," and "Nnn." Doing so, you might note how similar the sounds are to the chants of Tibetan and Gregorian monks as well as the songs of indigenous people found around the world. Of course, those songs and chants include consonants because they are meaningful sentences. You can add consonants too but be cognizant that the vagal nerve stimulating aspects of the chants and songs come from the sustained vibrations. To get a sense of the sounds, I invite you to download the primary sound mp3 at: https://richardlhaight.com/primarysounds/

Hopefully, you can feel the depth of these sounds from the little experience you have had from this chapter. Know that the depth of primary sounds runs still deeper. Beyond the practical contributions to our language and health, we find that vocalizing primary sounds in the right way for a long enough time can lead people into visionary states that transcend the self, states that even an atheist would be hard pressed to describe as anything other than transcendent. You cannot get that effect from secondary sounds or consonants.

Let's look at the known science regarding primary sounds, the breath, the vagal nerve, and how it all affects our health and awareness.

The vagal nerve, which connects the brain stem to the vital organs, also connects with the posterior wall of the external auditory canal, the lower part of the eardrum's membrane as well as to the middle ear ("Vagus Nerve"). Chanting primary sounds produces a measurable increase in the strength of the vagal response, which is determined by heart rate variation.

The greater the heart rate variation between breathing in and breathing out, the healthier is the vagal tone. When we breathe in before making the "Ah" sound, for example, the heart rate will elevate. Then as we exhale while producing the sound, our heart rate measurably drops. Producing primary sounds in a mantra-like fashion strengthens vagal tone. Not only does vagal tone improve through this exercise, but the limbic system calms. The limbic system is the emotional center of the brain. Vagal stimulation through any means stabilizes our emotions, which allows us more inner clarity.

If we were to measure brain waves before, during, and after chanting primary sounds, we could see that the brain shifts from a beta wave, thinking, aiming, stress-inducing state, into alpha wave, which is a restorative state. Watching TV would also put us into alpha wave state. The difference is that with vagal toning we are in a highly aware, meditated state as compared to TV watching, which is an unaware state.

Chapter 5

Sound Dimensions

Each primary sound has a distinct resonance, shape, and vibrational direction that can be felt in the body. The more skillful you are at vocalizing these sounds from deep within the body, the more obvious are the shapes, dimensions, and directional flows of each sound. To get a basic sense of the distinct dimensionality of each sound, we can vocalize them in succession, without stopping between sounds.

Here is how to feel the nature of each sound:

1. Sit up or stand straight but comfortably.
2. Relax the body and defocus the mind while feeling the entire physical body.
3. Begin vocalizing "Ah" while feeling the vibrations in the body for a few seconds. Note the shape and direction of vibrational travel.

4. Shift the sound to "Ee" for a few seconds and note the vibrational change in shape as compared to making the "Ah" sound. Notice the direction that the sound travels.
5. Continuing, change the sound to "Ew" for a brief duration. Feel and note the shape and direction of sound travel as compared to the "Ee" sound.
6. Shift into the "Eh" sound and note the change, the shape, and the travel of the sound.
7. Change to the "Oh" sound and feel its qualities.
8. Make the "Mmm" sound and note its nature.
9. Finally, produce the "Nnn" sound and feel its dimensions.

To get a sense of them, produce them all in one breath, while feeling the change between them.

"Ah"
"Ee"
"Ew"
"Eh"
"Oh"
"Mmm"
"Nnn"

If you have not already done so, I invite you to download the primary sound mp3 at: https://richardlhaight.com/primarysounds/

By now you can see and clearly feel the differences in sound dimension between each of these primary vocalizations. You probably noticed that the "Ah" sound travels down the body, the "Ee" sound makes a narrow but wide almost horizontal disk-like shape from the upper chest or throat. The "Ew" sound travels up in a conical shape, while the "Eh" sound aims that conical shape to the fore. The "Oh" sound is a spherical sound that moves away from its origin in every direction equally. By contrast, the "Mmm" sound is also spherical but small by comparison to the "Oh" sound. What shape is the "Nnn" sound?

If at first you feel unsure of the dimensions of the sound, do not be too concerned, for developing bodily awareness and sensitivity is part of the benefit of primary sound exercises. It may take a little practice before you clearly sense the dimensions of the sounds and develop an understanding of how they travel. I recommend practicing each sound a little each day to get a feel for it.

During your practice, notice any sounds that feel difficult to produce from deep within the body. Most people, when they first begin chanting primary sounds, create the sounds heavily from the throat, which makes the pitch higher than is ideal for the practice. To help produce the sounds from deeper within the body, place your hands over the diaphragm, the soft area just below your breastbone, so you can feel that area a little more acutely. Try to produce the sounds from that area. Opening the mouth a little wider drops the pitch of the sound so that you feel it lower in the body.

Don't worry too much about producing perfect sounds. The purpose of the practice is not to improve your singing voice or to perform for others. Refinement of the sounds will come with practice. The most important thing is to relax, feel, and enjoy the process, for to do otherwise does not allow for the meditative benefits of the practice.

Chapter 6

Sound Therapy

You might have noticed while producing the different sounds that the body felt positive while producing certain sounds and somewhat averse to producing other sounds. Still other sounds felt neutral. Take note of the sounds that feel especially good to your body, for when you produce those sounds it is quite beneficial to your health.

To gain the maximum health benefits from these sounds, direct your efforts to producing the sounds which create the most positive feelings in the body as you make them. Try each sound while feeling the body's response– "Ah," "Ee," "Ew," "Eh," "Oh," "Mmm" and "Nnn".

The sound that is therapeutic at this time will feel somehow right or fulfilling to your body. Take note of that sound, for you will be making use of it. You also want to know which sound your body is currently feeling averse to. Feeling for these two extremes will help to dial in your physical sensitivity and awareness, which will aid you in later exercises.

From testing, I have found that no one sound is right for everyone. I have also realized that our bodies are constantly changing, so the sound that felt great to the body this morning might not be the right one at noon or at night. The key is to make the sounds entirely without expectation, feeling each before selecting the right one for the moment. Set a timer to five minutes and enjoy vocalizing the therapeutic sound.

As you can probably see from practicing these sounds even a little, the vocalizations will tone your vagal nerve and put you into a meditative state of mind very quickly, but another reason supports use of the practice: the development of subconscious awareness.

If we look at the mind as an ocean, which is a typical metaphor for mind and consciousness, we could consider the surface as representing the mind. It is full of change and turmoil. The deeper we dive below the surface, which represents the subconscious, the more clarity and awareness we find. The way to dive deeper is through feeling. As we practice feeling the differences between the sounds, and especially how those sounds feel to our bodies on a therapeutic level, the more aware we become of the subconscious mind, which has its own currents.

The truest level of awareness is found beneath all currents. When that level is reached and sustained throughout daily life, we call it total embodiment. Before we can live our lives at that depth of awareness, we need to first become consciously aware of the currents between the surface and the stillness. Practicing with the aim of developing inner sensitivity is the secret to purposefully diving deeper into the ocean of the subconscious.

To aid you in your practice we can further refine each sound by trying each one in its low and high pitch form and then noting exactly which pitch feels right for your body at this time. Let's imagine you tested all the primary sounds and found that in this moment the "Ah" sound feels exactly right. To dial the exact pitch in for the "Ah" sound you could start out producing it with as low a pitch as you can, which will require your mouth to be fully open with the sound coming from your diaphragm. As you produce the sound, slowly move the origin of the sound up toward the throat. If you are able to do this, the pitch of the "Ah" should increase significantly. As you slowly raise the pitch, notice exactly which pitch feels most therapeutic for your body in the moment.

Once you have a sense for which sound and pitch seem most beneficial right now, see if you can also identify the sound and pitch to which your body feels most averse. Practicing in this way will increase your awareness and physical sensitivity over time and can allow a kind of conscious communication with the subconscious mind.

Once you find both the therapeutic and the adverse sounds, make sure you finish your practice working on the sound that produced the greatest therapeutic benefit to your body. Always leave on a positive note if you can.

Part III

Basic Pressure Training

You have now learned several training tools to improve your health, physical sensitivity, and meditative awareness. In Part III, you are going to learn a powerful tool which will without doubt challenge your abilities.

If you are a beginner, the first thought you might have is that you are not ready for a challenge. Banish that thought as quickly as it arises, for it does not reflect the truth. The pressure training described in Part III might overwhelm you the first few times you try it, but that will be the case regardless of your meditative ability.

What will happen is this: the first few times, you will notice feeling overwhelmed, but shortly thereafter you will see rapid improvement, and taking note of that improvement will encourage the practice of pressure training.

The pressure training that we will use is born of an ancient religious practice known as purification by water. For our purposes, we strip away all religious elements so that we can work purely with the principles of the practice. Adhering to the principles will turn purification by water into a powerful awareness training tool.

Once we learn the basic method, we will explore proper breathing as it relates to the practice as well as variations to the method that will allow you to make appropriate adjustments according to your circumstances each day. Once we learn the variations, we will discuss health-related issues that may require slight modifications to allow for productive, safe practice.

Finally, we will learn to use a powerful progress assessment tool derived from primary sounds that will accurately reveal where you are in your training, so you can increase the difficulty level appropriately.

Chapter 7

Purification by Water

Purification by water can be found in almost every culture and religion around the world. For example, John the Baptist, a Jewish prophet in the time of Jesus, is described in the Bible as baptizing people by immersing them in river water as a central sacrament to his messianic teachings. It is written that Jesus went to John to be baptized before he began his ministry. Of course, baptism still thrives today in most Christian traditions, but baptism as it is typically practiced now is not exactly as it was at the time of John.

The tradition of purification by water, known as *tvilah* in Judaism, long predates John the Baptist, and is found in the Law of Moses, written over a thousand years before John's mission. The *tvilah* ritual requires that the individual be immersed in a natural collection of water, called a *mikveh.* Through immersion in water, it is said that the individual is restored to "purity." The ritual serves to purify someone who converts to Judaism, prior to entering the Holy Temple, or after having touched a corpse, for example.

In Japanese culture, a similar practice, known as *misogi* (禊), translates into English as "to perform ablution." In the Shinto tradition *misogi* means to wash away impurities with water and is performed under a waterfall. In fact, to this day people practice *misogi* at waterfalls found at large Buddhist temples or Shinto shrines around the country.

The practice is typically performed by stripping off one's clothing down to the underwear. While praying, the individual wades out under the waterfall and remains there for as long as they can with the intention of maintaining their conviction to release spiritual impurities, or to pray for others.

Due to the focus on ritualistic and religious elements and the perception that these practices are born of ancient superstitions, the practical elements of purification by water have largely been forgotten. Losing track of the underlying principle is understandable when we consider that purification by water was used as a tool of exorcism in many religions around the world. If one does not believe in spirits, exorcism makes no sense, and by association, neither does purification by water.

Unfortunately, by dismissing this practice, we in the modern world have largely relegated one of the most essential practices for our health and well-being to the bin of superstition. The idea of washing away evil spirits may seem absurd to the secular way of thinking, but if we consider what one experiences when intentionally stepping under a cold waterfall for the purpose of purification, the idea of washing away evil spirits becomes easier to grasp. Allow me to explain.

Ancient peoples worldwide thought of differing emotional states as being spirits. The basic idea was that the state of clarity represented the true or pure you, the spark of the divine. Emotions that cause confusion or lead to poor behavior or unhealthy thinking were not considered the true self, but instead spirits that had temporarily possessed the person. In modern terms, we might categorize extreme emotional states as temporary insanity.

We have all experienced emotional outbursts and the suffering caused by hasty words or actions taken while in an unclear state. Most of us would assume we are only talking about anger and haste, but any form of emotionally stimulated lack of clarity could count as a spirit possession by the old way of thinking.

Consider for example the urge that compels you to buy that new car or eat that ice cream when you know you shouldn't. Or think about the emotional biases that cause people to be blind to facts that may be staring them in the face. You might choose to wash away those spirits if you could.

Chapter 8

Facing the Water

As we discussed in the last chapter, the ancients thought that immersion into natural water with the intention to purify oneself exorcised negative spirits. From that description, we can see that two of the elements at play for the ancients may not apply to us–the type of water and the belief in spirits. As our life circumstances differ markedly from those of the ancients, we need to know if those elements apply to us or not.

Regarding the requirement for natural water–we should recall that the ancients did not have running water in their homes. Natural water, to them, was water that ran through rivers, creeks, oceans, et cetera, i.e., water that was well below body temperature.

Although you can't access a river from within your home, you can use the shower. The only question is whether taking a cold shower provides the purifying effect for us or not. We also need to know if belief in spirits is required to gain the benefits of purification by water. If your emotional state clears because of taking an intentional cold shower, then you will know that the basic idea of purification by water is useful. To answer either question will require your direct experience with an intentional cold shower. Let's test the theory by conducting an experiment.

Note: if you have a heart condition or are otherwise in poor health, please consult your health practitioner before conducting this experiment.

Wait until you feel negative or otherwise emotional, then head into your bathroom, strip off your clothes, and step into a stream of the coldest water your shower can provide with the intention that the shocking embrace of the cold water washes away the negativity.

Be sure to stand completely under the flowing water for at least a minute. Direct the water to your face, over your head, chest and back. Do not attempt to escape the stream in any way. In fact, intentionally direct the water to the places that cause your breathing to constrict the most. Breathe with the aim of relaxing into the experience. Intentionally release negativity with your breath. After one minute, turn off the water, step out of the shower, and dry your body.

How do you feel?

The first thing you will likely notice is your body feels alive, stimulated as compared to before entering the shower. Notice also your experiential state has been cleansed, such that you feel comparatively good physically, mentally, and emotionally. Simply put, you feel better, think more clearly, and have more energy. To the thinking of the ancients, you have been purified.

Hopefully, after your experience with the cold shower, the idea of purification by water no longer seems so absurd. If you had no scientific explanation to rely on, you too would likely describe yourself as having been cleansed of an impure spirit.

Unfortunately, many of the religions that practice these rituals do not teach, and maybe do not know, the original healthful practice that engendered their rituals. If they did, the practice of purification by water would be a normal part of people's life routine, not a once a year or once in a lifetime ritual.

For our purposes, we will set aside all religious associations and stick with the practical benefits that we get from the taking intentional cold showers, which are that you feel much better physically, mentally, and emotionally. With experience, you will notice you are more capable, more productive, more aware, more energetic on days that you take cold showers than you are on days when you skipped the cold shower.

Some people think that taking a cold shower is an extreme activity because it feels so shocking. Such thoughts come from a modernized perspective where we are used to having easy access to heated water every time we shower or bathe. But heated water was not what our bodies evolved with. In fact, up until very recently, bathing in cold water was just a normal part of hygiene, done all year-round.

With the invention of farming, humans began to live more sedentary lifestyles. Eventually we began heating water for bathing. Heated water then became the norm, and our bodies have weakened as a result.

As you may recall, in Part I we discussed the beneficial effects that TEM training has on the brain and on the body through vagal stimulation. With each cold shower experience, your vagal nerve will be highly stimulated, which will increase your heart rate variation, a very positive health outcome. Because of intense vagal stimulation, bodily inflammation will reduce, so your overall health will likely improve.

With each cold shower, you are exercising your circulatory system, specifically the heart and the muscles in the walls of the blood vessels, which will improve their capacity to regulate blood pressure throughout your body. Furthermore, a cold shower will exercise the mitochondria in your cells, making them more efficient. The cells that have insufficient mitochondria will die off to be replaced by healthier cells. The net effect is a cellular pruning that will allow more energy so your body is in better overall health than it would be otherwise. Finally, as you take on the challenge of the cold shower experience, you will discover you are better able to take on other challenges you might have been avoiding.

To summarize, the result of daily cold showers is a healthier heart, a more toned nervous system, a better immune system, a stronger circulatory system, and healthier cells. In ancient times those systems had to be robust just to survive. In modern times, we can get by without having a strong body, but our quality of life suffers.

No matter who you are or what your intention, taking cold showers can afford certain benefits. That said, if your intention is right, which is to be more meditatively aware, the benefits will extend further. Challenging emotional inertia with a cold shower will greatly enhance your awareness and meditative abilities under any kind of pressure, including those of daily life.

Before we get to that type of training, let's cover some cold shower safety protocols.

Who should not take cold showers?

Although most physicians warn individuals with heart conditions to avoid cold water immersion (think ice baths), there is little written about the dangers of a cold shower. That said, for individuals who have severely compromised health, at the end of this chapter I include a step-up system that will allow your body to acclimate to cold showers more slowly, if you and your doctor approve.

If you suspect you have a condition that may not be compatible with taking cold showers, please read through this entire chapter before attempting a cold shower. Even people who are generally healthy will want to use some aspects of that system on days when they are not feeling well.

Breath of Fire

How we breathe in the first minute of a cold shower makes a big difference as to how long we can stay in there. As beginners, we may notice that our breathing becomes convulsive and erratic when the cold water first hits our skin. Or we may be tempted to hold our breath as a response to a stressful situation. With that awareness in mind, we can use the shower experience to learn how to guide our breathing toward stability.

To get our breathing under control in a cold shower scenario, all that is required is to intentionally surf the convulsive breathing into rapid, full, powerful inhales and exhales. Doing so will rapidly tone your vagal nerve, oxygenize your blood and potentially even raise your body temperature.

This type of breathing has been codified by Tibetan monks and is commonly referred to as Breath of Fire. The method is so named because if done properly, a master practitioner can demonstrably raise their body temperature even when sitting naked on ice. Properly understood, Breath of Fire is not exactly a technique so much as a conscious surfing of what the body naturally does when exposed to sudden cold. Of course, people tend to overcomplicate and ritualize things that are quite simple. For our purposes with the shower, there is no need to complicate Breath of Fire. When you start the cold shower, if your breathing is convulsive, you could use Breath of Fire to get the breathing under control again.

First Training Shower

Note: for safety, always set a timer for 10 minutes to remind you to get out before hypothermia sets in.

To get the maximum benefit of a cold shower, do it first thing in the morning after using the toilet. With as little thought as possible, strip off your clothes, step into the shower, and if you can get yourself to do it, position yourself fully under the faucet and turn the water on to the strongest, coldest setting possible.

As the water envelops your body, notice any flinch responses or unstable breathing. Use the first minute to try to get your breathing under control using Breath of Fire, while directing the flow of the water directly to the places that stimulate the most breathing tension.

Once past the first minute, aim to stay in the cold shower for as long as you can, but no more than 10 minutes. We do not want the body's core temperature to drop into hypothermia, which can be a life-threatening condition.

If you are able to get your breathing under control in the first minute, remaining in the shower for longer will not be so difficult. If, however, your breathing does not smooth out, the challenge of the shower will be overwhelming, and you may be unable to stay in the shower beyond a minute. If that happens, don't beat yourself up about it. With daily practice, you'll soon find you can easily do one minute.

Note: if you have trouble warming up or you feel a burning sensation after the shower, it means your core body temperature has dropped a bit, something that we want to avoid. Try reducing the time in the shower a bit until those symptoms no longer show.

Gradual Approach

If you experience heavy resistance to stepping fully into the cold shower stream, you can take it one step at a time, via a more gradual approach. Here is how you might proceed.

Imagine you are wading into a river to bathe, as you would have done in ancient times. Quite naturally, your feet enter the cold water first. As you wade in deeper, the water rises up your legs, to your crotch, then your lower abdomen before you finally take the plunge and dive under the water.

With that scenario as our guide, you might direct the shower stream first to your feet, then gradually up your legs, to your crotch, then to your lower abdomen. You might also direct the spray up your arms before finally aiming the stream at your torso, face, head, shoulders, and down your back.

Once past the first minute, aim to stay in the cold shower for up to 10 minutes, but no longer. Again, the aim for the first minute is to get the breath under control and to relax into the cold water experience. If your breathing does not smooth out, the challenge of the shower will be overwhelming, and you may be unable to remain in the cold spray for long. In that case, you are wise to exit early because your body will not regulate temperature well when the breathing is highly erratic.

If you can't remain in the shower, do not berate yourself about it. You'll get the hang of it soon. Regardless of how long you remained there, mentally note the time you were in there, and, if you were able to regulate your breathing, roughly how long it took to smooth it out.

Once your shower is complete, immediately dry yourself. Air drying after a cold shower is ill-advised for beginners as the body can rapidly lose core temperature, resulting in hypothermia, a dangerous and potentially life-threatening condition.

The Sink Method

For individuals who are in ill health but would like to challenge themselves with the cold, there is a much gentler way. The sink method will benefit the heart without putting it in danger. To be sure, check with your health practitioner before you proceed with this method.

As the vagal nerve connects to our face and neck, we can stimulate it and positively affect the rest of our body by pouring cold water over our head, neck and face. I use this method on days when my health feels mildly compromised.

Put your head under the sink faucet and run cold water over your head. Use your hand to direct the faucet water over your face and neck. Keep up this process for at least a minute. When done with the head, face, and neck, run the cold water over your arms.

Once you are done with the water, hold your head above the sink for a few minutes to let the water drip off and be exposed to the air in the room. Notice your breathing. You might note you have breath releases every now and again, where your body naturally sucks in a large breath and releases it in an invigorating way. Dry yourself and go about your day.

If you find that the water temperature from the tap is not enough of a challenge, you could fill a bucket or a large bowl with water and then add enough ice to cover the entire surface of the water about 10 minutes prior to your sink adventure. That should give enough time for the water temperature to drop significantly. Remove the ice and dump the water over your head in one move, if possible. Follow this with the sink method as prescribed above.

Final note: your sink counter can become a watery mess with this method, which I do not find a problem. If you wanted you could use this method in the shower instead, if you have a detachable shower head.

Q & A about cold showers

Question: I find it hard to clean my body while taking a cold shower, so I also take warm showers. It seems like a waste of water to do both.

Answer: The cold showers work fine for cleaning the body, but you would need to do it the old way using a rough cloth to exfoliate the skin. In this way, you remove the dead skin but keep the healthy oils. You may find your skin does not dry out so easily this way and is healthier than it would be if you always used soap. Regarding cleaning the hair, that too can be done with a cold shower and without soap, but it takes some months of hard work rebalancing your scalp and pore health. As few people would be willing to do what is required, and as that aspect does not pertain much to this book, I will skip it here.

Question: Do I need to take cold showers to awaken?

Answer: What is required depends on the individual. That said, the inner force that wants to avoid the discomfort of the cold shower may be the very thing that is preventing what may be described as awakening. In any case, to awaken, if that is your aim, it requires a softening of resistance to change, challenges, and discomfort. Cold showers will help you to do that.

Question: Can cold showers make you sick?

Answer: So many of us were told, "Put your coat on or you'll catch your death of cold! Stay out of the rain or you'll get sick." You don't get a cold from being cold. A cold comes from a virus, not from the temperature. That said, if your immune system is severely compromised and you have the cold virus, then you could get sick. The best way to remain healthy is to strengthen the immune system. To do that, one must challenge the immune system. The concept is no different from lifting weights for the purpose of becoming stronger. To summarize, managed exposure to cold and other pressures is beneficial to overall health.

Question: Will you get hypothermia if you take cold showers in the winter?

Answer: You can get hypothermia in any temperature below your body temperature. People get hypothermia after being in 65-degree Fahrenheit temperatures for too long. Defense against hypothermia depends largely on your health. The key to avoiding hypothermia after cold exposure is to heat your body back up. You can do that with warm water, by putting on sufficient dry clothing, drinking a warm beverage, et cetera.

Chapter 9

Flowing with Health Issues

As we are working with cold exposure, we need to be cognizant of possible disorders than can complicate our training–most notably, Raynaud's Syndrome and associated autoimmune disorders. If you do not suffer from autoimmune disorders, feel free to skip to the next chapter.

Raynaud's Syndrome is a circulatory disorder that causes decreased blood flow to the fingers, but it can also affect the toes, knees, nipples, ears, nose, or lips. According to Johns Hopkins Hospital's Rheumatology department, Raynaud's symptoms are due to spasms of blood vessels in those listed areas. The spasms are triggered by exposure to cold, stress, or emotional upset.

Raynaud's affects about four percent of the population. The most common form of Raynaud's typically shows in people between ages of 15 and 30 and most commonly in females.

When Raynaud's shows up in people older than 30, it is typically linked to other disorders such as autoimmune or connective tissue diseases like lupus, scleroderma, CREST syndrome, Buerger's disease, Sjögren's syndrome, rheumatoid arthritis, occlusive vascular disease, polymyositis, blood disorders, thyroid disorders, and pulmonary hypertension. Although those links are common, the true cause of Raynaud's is still unknown.

The symptoms of Raynaud's can vary a bit from person to person, but there are common elements. The first and most common symptom is fingers that turn pale or white, then blue, when exposed to cold. This symptom is often accompanied by numbness and pain. Raynaud's can also express during stress or emotional upset. Another symptom is hands that swell and feel painful when warmed. When the hands are warmed, they eventually turn red. Warming typically takes minutes, but it can, in rare cases, take hours for proper circulation to return to the affected areas. In severe cases, sores can form on the finger pads, which can easily lead to infection and possibly gangrene that can, in rare situations, require amputation.

According to the Johns Hopkins Medical School's website, a number of factors can increase the risk of developing Raynaud's; namely, connective tissue or autoimmune disease, chemical exposure, cigarette smoking, injury or trauma, repetitive actions such as typing or use of vibrating tools such as chainsaws and jackhammers, and the side effects from certain medicines ("Raynaud's Phenomenon").

Raynaud's management typically includes avoiding stressors that stimulate it, such as cold, stress, or emotional upset. If you have Raynaud's, you are advised to dress warmly and avoid smoking. Caffeine, estrogen, and nonselective beta-blockers are often listed as aggravating factors, but evidence is still insufficient to be sure they should be avoided (Wigley and Flavahan).

I have personal experience with Raynaud's, as does one of my siblings. In my case, it began when I was older, apparently as a complication of an autoimmune disorder that expressed as rheumatoid arthritis in my spine. My doctor said that this arthritis was most likely stimulated by a horse accident when I was 17, an event that crushed my spine like an accordion.

As I entered my forties, the first symptoms of Raynaud's began to show in my fingers, which would go colorless and numb when I washed my hands in cold water or when I was out in cold air. Raynaud's became a learning opportunity. I could not take a cold bath, something I used to enjoy, so I switched to modified cold showers. If you have Raynaud's, and your doctor approves, there are some easy adjustments you can use to take cold showers.

If cold showers stimulate Raynaud's, the trick is to first fill up the bathtub with warm water and then stand in that warm water while taking the cold shower. Once the shower is complete, lie down in the warm bath to warm the core back up.

I began taking bodily inflammation seriously and used all my knowledge and awareness to overcome the issue. I realize that everything I was doing was profoundly helpful and anti-inflammatory: vagal breathing, meditating, chanting, cold water showers, an anti-inflammatory diet, all had important impacts. Practiced persistently, you've got a cutting-edge protocol that may prevent or reduce symptoms of Raynaud's and associated inflammatory disorders.

Maintaining this protocol for a while, I found that I could take the cold showers without experiencing Raynaud's symptoms. If, however, I consumed any caffeine, the symptoms would return. Caffeine, much like tobacco, is a vasoconstrictor. Testing it again and again, I found a perfect correlation between consuming caffeine and experiencing Raynaud's symptoms from cold exposure.

Typically, it took three to four days of abstaining from caffeine to no longer have the Raynaud's reaction when in the cold shower. Even decaffeinated coffee and tea would elicit the reaction because there is no way to entirely remove caffeine. And who knows, there may be other substances in coffee that did not suit my body.

After several years of maintaining a strong anti-inflammatory routine, I find I can drink a cup of caffeinated coffee or tea and take a cold shower without a Raynaud's response; however, a cold bath will reveal the symptoms. Of course, what I am sharing about my personal experience may or may not apply to other people's health conditions, but scientific research does show that all of the above mentioned practices have anti-inflammatory and immune regulating benefits, so I hope you find them to be as helpful as I do.

Many of my students who have taken the challenge of incorporating TEM practices into their lives have reported remarkable health improvements. I suspect that if you explore the tools you have been offered here and dial in your diet, you may find that Raynaud's as well as many other autoimmune disorders, subside or disappear entirely from your life. Even for people who do not recognize that they have autoimmune issues, these changes might bring about a reduction or elimination of joint creaks, stiff necks, and tight shoulders.

As for cold showers, if you have health conditions that make you prone to adverse reactions, try taking them while standing in hot or warm bath water, so that as soon as the shower is complete, you can sink into the warm bath to rapidly heat up your core temperature, which will get blood back into the ill-affected areas.

If your Raynaud's reaction manifests so extremely that even the warm bath option does not work for you, you may find the following modification to the protocol helpful. We can use our body for thermal storage to prevent the Raynaud's response while in the cold shower. The way to do this is to first fill up the bath with hot water and bathe until your body is filled with heat.

Once the body battery is charged with heat, stand up in the warm water and turn on the cold shower. Doing this, you will find that the cold is not nearly so shocking because your body is radiating such heat. The stored energy will have warmed your blood, which will likely keep your circulatory system from blocking blood flow to the extremities.

Once you are finished with the shower, you might find you are still warm. If not, you could always lie back down in the bath to warm back up.

This protocol should keep you safe from severe Raynaud's reactions as you correct your health over time. Before too long, you may find you no longer need the pre-bath ritual, and with further practice, you may discover you can safely skip the post-bath as well.

Other disabilities

If you suffer from another health condition that prevents safe applications of cold showers, here is another approach that may work well for you.

Using your sink or a bucket of cold water, wet a washcloth and use it to spread the cold water over your body. If, for example, you were in a wheelchair, you could remove your shirt, socks, and pull up your pant legs to expose your lower legs. Wipe the wet towel over the exposed areas, including your face and neck.

You will notice that the washcloth quickly becomes warm from your body heat, so you will want to continually re-wet it with cold water as you go about wiping your body. With each application of cold, you may notice your nervous system responds with a bit of tension. That is fine.

Once you have wet your body, the challenge will be to allow the body to air dry. Air drying can quickly drop your body temperature, so, air drying may be ill-advised for individuals who experience strong Raynaud's symptoms. Any resulting Raynaud's symptoms are a good indicator if you need to skip the airdrying.

As you air dry, you will likely notice that the nipples tighten. A bit of shivering is also to be expected, but once the shivering becomes so strong that your teeth start to chatter, be sure to towel off, put your clothes back on, and do what you can to reheat your body.

Practicing in this way for months, you are likely to notice your body is able to relax more when the cold cloth touches the skin. It will not begin shivering so quickly. You will be able to air dry longer, and your body will warm up quicker. These are all important signs of improvement!

Chapter 10

Measuring Progress

At this point in our training, you will note little difference between what we are doing and what other cold enthusiasts are doing. All forms of cold training can be beneficial if practiced safely. As we progress, you will start to see a certain, but critical divergence in the methodology. All TEM training tools are meant to help us be clear and capable in every moment of our lives, which means to have vibrant, meditative awareness at all times, as would be the aim of a master Samurai.

The Samurai Mindset

Imagine you are a Samurai warrior, whose life and capacity to serve and protect depends on a sustained awareness even under tremendous pressure. Suppose you must cross a near freezing river while on duty. Would you flinch from the cold? Would your breathing become spasmodic? If you were a Samurai worth his stipend, no. If you had not trained yourself properly, you would struggle with the river, and your master, seeing your struggle, would probably remove you from his employment because while flinching and breathing spasmodically, you are certainly not aware or capable of effective service.

To train the body and mind to be less reactive, less prone to flinch, conscientious Samurai made use of cold training, sometimes under waterfalls, but often at home or out in the field with buckets of cold water upon rising from sleep. Their aim was not only to condition the body and mind to be less flinch prone, but also to wake up sharp and capable, ready for action.

One of the key traits of a master Samurai was that he was always seeking to measure his abilities, to be sure of his current capacity and condition. Honoring that mindset, I will provide you with a number of powerful tools to measure your current capacity and your progress.

You can probably relate to the frustration people feel when they are unable to see clear progress from their efforts, which might make them more prone to quit. If you had a measuring device that clearly demonstrated your improvement, you would be far more likely to continue your training.

The great thing about the body is that it does not lie. No matter how aware we might like to imagine ourselves to be, when placed under pressure, the breathing and circulatory system will tell the truth. So let us swallow our pride and take advantage of that fact by applying a measuring device to our cold water training that will demonstrate our body's capacity to breathe smoothly when exposed to the sudden cold.

Measuring Progress through Primary Sounds

As I said in the introduction to Part III, the key to making rapid progress is pacing yourself properly as an individual. If you try to keep a pace that I might recommend, and you are the average person, it will likely work out alright for you; but if you are outside the norm, the pace will be inappropriate to you. Rather than attempting to conform to a one-size-fits-all pace, it would be much better if you could accurately find your own pacing.

We can use primary sounds for that purpose. Here is how it works. Right before entering the shower, take a full breath and begin loudly vocalizing the primary sounds of "Ah" to get a baseline for the stability of the sound when not under pressure. Continue chanting the sound until your lungs are empty. That will give a general sense of how loud, smooth, and long you can sustain the sound from one breath when not under pressure.

Be sure you open your mouth enough that the sound resonates sufficiently, but don't blast it out so loud that it annoys family members. You might consider informing them of this practice before you do it, so as not to surprise anyone.

Now that you have your baseline for your primary sound, enter the shower, take another breath, and begin producing your sound. Immediately turn on the water and aim it to run over your head, chest, and back, especially the areas that are most challenging.

Notice any wavering of the primary sound. Typically, beginners find that they can't maintain a chant because their lungs are spasming too much to produce a controlled sound. If you are new to cold showers, you are likely unable to produce the sound under pressure exactly as you could prior to the water exposure. Do not fret, because now you know your current capacity as compared to where you want it to be, which is exactly as it was before you started the shower. Again, your breathing reflects the capacity of the physical body to remain clear and capable under pressure.

Regardless of how you performed the first time you used primary sounds to assess your capacity, we are going to want improvement. With that in mind, each day aim to make the same full bodied, lengthy sounds in the cold shower as you did prior to taking the cold shower.

From this exercise, you will notice that any lung contractions can be easily heard and felt when chanting. Notice too that when these contractions happen, even if they are small, you are not able to produce the sound as fully or as long as you could when you were not under pressure.

People who are more acclimated to cold might be able to produce a primary sound, but not quite as smoothly as they could before the shower. Practicing primary sounds with each cold shower over a period of days will typically demonstrate obvious improvement. Such improvement is not just in your ability to produce a sound, but in your body's capacity to handle stress while remaining aware and capable, something that will be helpful in every stressful moment of your life!

After a few weeks, you may find you can make a perfect "Ah," sound. The next challenge would be to try the "Oh" sound. If you can produce that sound well too, then move on to the "Mmm" sound and see how that goes. Once that sound is mastered, move on to the "Eh" sound. Continuing in this way, as you have mastered each sound, move to the next. After Eh, try the "Ew" and "Ee" sounds to find which is the next proper challenge. Work your way through the sounds until you are left with your last sound. Aim to master that sound. Within a few weeks to a month, you will likely find you can flawlessly or near flawlessly produce all of these sounds in a cold shower.

To summarize, when chanting, the subtle shifts in breathing show up in the sound and in the pressure of our diaphragmatic contractions, so you can much more easily hear and feel them. The sound makes obvious what was otherwise obscure.

Part IV

Training the Mind

For the vast majority of us, whether we recognize it or not, our own mind is our greatest obstacle. With your training, you will soon recognize how much your mind might be resisting your wise aims or how often it leads you astray through unhealthy urges and compulsions.

When we really pay attention to what is happening with our thoughts and emotions, we can't help but admit that we are not in fact in control of our lives. If we make a list of all healthy things that we are determined to do with our lives, we might discover that we actually follow through on but a few of those aims. Even getting the aims of a single day to manifest in our experience can seem like herding cats. Or, to consider the problem from another angle, we might create a list of unhealthy pleasures that we wish to avoid, only to find that our urges and compulsions have led us to do many or all of them.

When we zoom out to take a year-long view of our life pattern, we might see that our healthy habit choices did not last nearly as long as we had intended and that we are living quite astray from the path that we had entered on New Year's Day. Maybe we don't even bother to make goals anymore.

We are wise to admit that we are not nearly as in charge of our lives as we want to think we are. The question is—what is in charge? In Part IV we begin an investigation into the nature of that which is in charge when we are not. Through our investigation, we will discover the ways in which that force resists our aims and how to navigate through those resistance attempts. With some basic inner navigation skills, we can mentor the mind to move in healthy directions, regardless of thoughts and feelings it conjures as it seeks to avoid doing what is beneficial, but uncomfortable.

Chapter 11

Dealing with Dread

After taking morning cold showers for a few days, you may notice some degree of physical or psychological resistance to morning showers. For many beginners of this practice, the morning wake-up carries with it the immediate dread of the cold shower. If you experience an inner groan and a strong desire to roll back over and go back to sleep, know you are not alone. In fact, these feelings are entirely normal early in the process.

To discover the true nature of these feelings, let's try changing things up a bit with our cold shower, specifically the timing. For the next few days, take your cold shower at a time of day when you are at or near peak energy. To figure out when you are most energetic, think about what time of the day you are typically lightest on your feet, the time when you are more willingly active.

Notice the degree of mental and physical resistance you feel prior to turning on the water. Notice also the degree of discomfort you feel in the shower and the length of time you are able to remain in the cold water as compared to when you take a cold shower first thing in the morning.

What you will likely notice is that when your body is energetic, you feel less resistance to the cold shower. The experience is less shocking, and you are able to remain in the cold water longer. This experiment demonstrates that when you have energy, you feel more motivated and are thus much more willing to take on uncomfortable challenges. Conversely, when your body is in a low-energy state, you feel less motivated and are prone to experience higher levels of physical and psychological resistance than you would otherwise.

To further exemplify the point, let's try another experiment, but this time first thing in the morning. Get up, head into the bathroom, and fill up the bathtub with hot water to your liking. Take care of your toilet necessities, and then when the bath is full, take off your clothes and get in. Remain in the warm water for five or ten minutes to fully warm up your core body temperature.

Once your body is charged with warmth, drain the water, stand up and get under the shower head. Turn it on to full cold and see how your body reacts. I'll bet this cold shower is much easier than you imagined it would be. The question is why.

We could look at the body as a rechargeable battery. When the body is full of energy, it is more capable of handling pressure with grace. When the battery is low, the body feels weak and delicate and will instinctively try to avoid pressures. The negative emotions that many of us feel in resistance to the present moment can often be banished when we simply strengthen the body in certain key ways.

By toning the nervous system, strengthening the muscles of the circulatory system, stimulating the generation of healthier cells, and making positive changes in the brain through neuroplasticity, we find that we have more energy and are more able to face intense pressure without wavering. Effectively, our battery has grown bigger and more efficient.

So that brings us back to the hot bath experiment. When you charged your body with hot water, the heat acted as a kind of insulation from the cold. If you remained in the cold long enough, your body would be drained of that extra heat, and your core temperature would begin to drop into hypothermia.

The key takeaway is that no matter how strong the body battery is, there will be limits to its tolerances, so we are wise to navigate the body's limits carefully. Early in the practice, the body energy may be comparatively feeble to the potential that can be achieved through regular daily training.

Coming back to daily life, if you pay attention to the times when you are most likely to feel frustrated, you will notice that it tends to happen when you are a little hungry or tired -- low energy. With that in mind, one of the most effective ways of reducing negative emotion and the often subsequent relationship strife is to strengthen the body's energy.

Of course, even if you train for more energy, you are still going to experience the mind's resistance games from time to time. This certainly happens to me. The mind's resistance process can be our ally, though, in that it helps us to be mindful of our energy.

The first thing to note when resistance arises is the mental narrative that accompanies it. "I hate these cold showers. I do not want to get in there." Then another voice says, "Yes, but I know it is good for me. I should get in there." This voice is countered by, "Yeah, but maybe I could skip today and do it tomorrow instead..."

Notice how one inner force aims to do what is healthy and another inner force seems aimed at avoiding discomfort. When we start closely observing inner forces, we realize that there are multitudes of them—it's a mess in there. We can grow more observant; we want to notice which forces predict our actions and inactions, for those forces represent our deepest patterns, many of which may need to be softened if we are to make real progress.

Each of these forces exists because they have been supported in some way. For instance, if we support the force that says, "I'll skip today and do it tomorrow instead," what we soon find is that the tomorrow where we actually follow through is harder and harder to come by, and before long we are no longer taking on the healthy challenge. And the more that we engage with challenges, the less power the resistive force has over us.

At first, though, the resistive force is going to fight like hell. And it will fight, and fight, and fight some more until it runs out of energy. If we allow the mind's attachment to comfortable inertia to dominate our decisions and actions, we are likely to feel guilt and lose self-respect later. The guilt is an attack on the self, and it is unhelpful. Or, instead of guilt, some people might blame the training system, thinking, "What sort of idiot thinks self-inflicted water-boarding is a viable life-improvement strategy?"

Okay, so maybe you didn't have that exact thought, but chances are your mind harbors some narrative that is unhelpfully critical of yourself or the training method. The first thing to know is that the resistance you feel is not wrong, nor is it right. If we experience intense resistance, it is unhelpful to deny what is in fact happening. We are not trying to perform some action "perfectly" on the first try; we are developing awareness through self-study. Right or wrong has little to do with the resistance. Be ready, without condemning yourself, to observe what is happening in your body and mind. And then keep going.

TEM training is not aimed merely at being able to handle cold with grace, but to be able to move gracefully through the myriad unhelpful forces that occur within and around us each day. Simply experiencing a cold shower willingly each morning, however disgraceful we may be feeling at the time, is helpful. So too is it helpful to wade through the many resistances your body and mind summon against the practice. It's all vital training that greatly improves the quality of your life, allowing unwavering awareness as you move through all manner of daily life difficulties.

Although actualizing such grace under pressure takes time, with practice the resistance does weaken. As the resistance weakens, the empowering force of awareness strengthens within us, making it much easier to tackle the challenges that further support well-being and awareness. "Myriad forces within us" might, at first glance, seem a little esoteric or woo-woo, but it accurately reflects what is actually happening in our brains constantly.

Each of the multitude of forces I talked about represent distinct but possibly networked neural pathways that have connected in association with our life pattern. The more we feed a neural pathway by agreeing with it and exercising it, the more the brain supplies that pathway with nutrients. Conversely, the less we use that neural pathway, the more the brain removes resources from that pathway to allocate to other pathways that are in use.

The most fundamental way that we strengthen an inner force is by identifying ourselves with that force. To exemplify the point, when you prepare to enter the shower and the voice in your head says, "I'll skip today and do it tomorrow instead," you might assume that voice was yours. If you were to explain the phenomena to a friend, you might say, "I was planning to take my cold shower, then just as I was about to take off my clothes, I thought to myself, 'I don't feel like taking a shower this morning, so I'll do it tomorrow instead."

As soon as you believe the thoughts and emotions which you experience to be you, you have supported those neural pathways by giving them the vital nutrient of identity. Instead, be curious. Try an experiment: what happens if, rather than identifying with thoughts and feelings, you merely notice the thoughts and feelings that the brain continually offers to your attention. Those thoughts and feelings only represent the existing neural pathways, mental/emotional ruts. They are not you.

An effective way to navigate those resistant neural patterns or attachments to unhelpful ways is to realize that they are simply brain habits that will change with persistent awareness. None of those forces represent the fundamental you, which existed prior to the development of those forces.

Over time, you will find that dis-identifying with thoughts and emotions is extremely helpful. That said, most of us, even if we do not consciously identify with unhelpful thoughts and feelings, still succumb to their influence sometimes.

Chapter 12

Mentoring the Mind

Resistive thoughts and feelings can be very persistent. To successfully transcend them, we do not want to avoid, deny, or get into a fight with resistive thoughts and feelings. The desire to avoid, deny, or fight itself represents a sympathetic nervous system reaction, known as the fight-or-flight response. Instead, we are seeking a way to study our internal workings and improve our responses without directing unkind thoughts toward ourselves.

The fight-or-flight response is a defensive peripheral nervous system response, which coincides with a high beta brain wave state that represents a disconnect from awareness. Disconnection is the antithesis of meditation and awareness. The fight-or-flight response triggers anxiety, disturbs breathing, and causes inflammation in the body, all of which will make your cold shower and daily life experience even more of a struggle.

The fight-or-flight response takes us away from primary awareness, not toward it. Instead of fighting, denying, or avoiding the thoughts and feelings, we are wise to soften them. The secret to softening is to take on the challenges you know you will in fact do today, rather than putting them off until tomorrow, a day that is likely to be skipped. Here is how to soften inner resistance.

When you notice the narrative, see if it feels like it is your voice. If it feels like your voice, it means you are identified with your thoughts and emotions, which means you think they are you. Pause, relax, and totally defocus your mind.

Once relaxed and defocused, try using the sink method you learned in Chapter 8. You may find you are able to use that method because it represents a pleasant step down from the threat of the cold shower, which the resistive inner force was so focused on avoiding.

Once your vagal nerve is stimulated from the sink method, consider the shower again. Would you be willing to get your feet wet? At this point, chances are you would because your body is already feeling somewhat better from vagal stimulation. Get in the shower and get your feet wet without any thought beyond that step.

Hold the cold spray on your feet for a bit and then ask yourself if you could try aiming the water at your lower legs. You'll likely discover you can. Now try your upper legs. Keep going until you finally reach a place where you are simply not willing to go any further. Most people will find that they are able to go all the way once they are a few steps into the process. If you hit what feels like an impenetrable blockage, stop, get out, and call it a day. The next day, do the same thing and see how far you can get. Chances are that within a week or two, you can take the full shower without nearly as much inner voice resistance.

The next step in dealing with the unhelpful inner force is to see if you can now directly enter the shower and speed up the process of the cold water exposure by making it a flowing progression instead of a step by step process. For example, maybe you spray the water onto your feet, and without stopping, slowly move upwards to your abdomen and then do your arms and your chest. Maybe you end up stopping before getting to your head. That's progress. Be thankful. Try again the next day. Before long, you will be able to fully immerse yourself in the water.

With persistence over a period of days or weeks, it will only take you 10-20 seconds to get the water up to your head. Once you get to that point, the next step is to see how long you can remain in the cold shower, being mindful to not exceed your current capacity. Stop before the resistance gets too strong. Eventually, you will wean yourself of gradual approaches. You'll simply walk decisively into the shower, turn it to full cold, and instantly immerse your body into the water, and you'll enjoy it.

The secret regarding the gradual approaches is to first get a little momentum in the right direction by doing what you know you can do in this moment. Once you have taken that initial step, check to see what else you are willing to do. More often than not, if you start out with something small, you will discover you are able to do a lot more than you anticipated at the outset. The reason for this is that as you go, you are neither feeding nor fighting the resistive mind, but instead, step by step, allowing your body and brain to adjust. As it adjusts, so too does the attitude.

The great thing about this strategy to resistance is that it also works well as a strategy for leading difficult children. If you tell a resistive child to do their chores, they might balk and simply not do it. But if you say, "You can either take out the trash or do the dishes–choose," more often than not, they will not resist because they feel empowered by the choice that they have been offered.

Offering a directed choice puts you in a position of a mentor and the child in a position of feeling empowered to choose. This process helps a resistive child build the neural pathways of respect, cooperation, good communication, and responsibility over time. So too does affording your body a choice regarding the path through the cold shower, or any other challenge for that matter. When the body feels empowered it becomes your ally. Sometimes the fastest way is the circuitous route.

Chapter 13

Mentoring the Body

As we discussed, cold shower training will churn up resistive inner forces. To make progress with your training and to improve the quality of your life, getting to know the various forms of resistance you might experience is extremely helpful. Everyone experiences resistance, so do not in the least get down on yourself when it occurs, as feeling bad about these feelings does not help. Feeling resistance is natural when we are breaking old unhealthy patterns and forging new, healthy ones.

To familiarize yourself with the forces of resistance, as you go through cold shower training, observe both the inner narrative and the body's feeling, because not all resistance comes in narrative form. Sometimes we may have no inner dialogue, but still feel physical resistance, much like your dog might try to resist getting into the bathtub if it has not been properly acclimated to taking baths.

An easy way to understand what I mean by physical resistance is to remember when you were a child trying to do something scary for the first time. Here's a vivid memory from my childhood, the lessons from which I am still learning. Hopefully, you can relate.

When I was a young boy living in the countryside, the neighborhood kids would often gather at a nearby stream. The older kids would jump across at a certain spot, but I was always afraid to do so. Even when I was determined to jump and sprinted toward it, at the last moment my body would stop. There was inner dialogue before initiating the sprint ("What if I don't make it?") and again after the fruitless sprint ("I'm such a coward") but never during the movement. At the last moment, my body froze, even though I was determined to jump. The body itself seemed afraid to make the jump.

I can clearly remember at that young age doing an experiment related to the creek jump. I measured out the width of the stream bed with a long stick and then marked that width on the ground with two sticks. I backed up and jumped safely over the space between them repeatedly. From that experiment, I knew for certain that I could jump that stream, but still my body would stop at the edge of the stream bed. Fear was controlling my body, and I needed to find a way of overcoming the fear so that elder boys would stop teasing me.

Eventually, I made that jump, but the way I did it was by walking to a narrower area of the creek that was not challenging to the older boys but was to me. I found that my body would jump that area without much resistance. In fact, I truly enjoyed the thrill of it. I worked my way up from there, and within a few days, I was jumping the area that my body initially resisted.

We all have things that we resist. Sometimes, we need to work our way up to a challenge. How long it takes to face a challenge is less important than constantly making progress as we work toward accomplishing the aim.

Ultimately, through conscientious training, we create an inner alliance of forces, so that when we have a healthy goal our bodies will follow through, sans resistance. When that happens, we experience incredible clarity, and we know we have established a trusting alliance with our bodies. Our bodies will then follow our wise aims even if the path feels uncomfortable.

Again, do not in the least concern yourself if it takes you a long time to get to the point where you can take a simple cold shower without resistance. Recognize that each of the micro-steps you took along the path challenged your body, stimulated your vagal nerve, strengthened the muscles in your vascular and arterial walls, and built up healthier cells with higher mitochondrial counts, all while repatterning your brain for greater awareness!

Even with a gradual protocol, some individuals may experience enough resistance that they can't even do the sink method on a certain day. For those individuals there is an even more gradual approach that I do not generally advise for healthy adults. That method is to get into the shower with the intention of first using lukewarm water and slowly turning it toward cold as you acclimate physically and mentally during the session. Over time, you will be able to apply gradually colder showers.

If you have no resistive mental narratives, but your body feels skittish or reluctant about the cold shower, you could take it in steps just as you did with narrative resistance. Signs of skittishness can be seen in avoidance body language. You might note your body just does not seem to want to face the shower, and this feeling may be present as soon as you awaken in the morning. Maybe your mind feels a certain dread or fear that then creates an avoidance desire such as wanting to go back to sleep or maybe desiring to change up your morning routine to postpone the shower. For example, instead of heading for the bathroom first thing, you turn to the kitchen to prepare a cup of tea or coffee. These are all avoidance strategies meant to postpone what you know is helpful but uncomfortable.

When you notice feelings of avoidance or skittishness, no matter how small the symptoms, even if there are no mental narratives, you have two productive choices. First, simply experience the feeling for a moment to get to know its presence, then defocus your mind and meditate yourself to calm awareness. Once calm and centered in awareness, get in touch with the energy or force within you that feels unconditional love and wants you to become stronger, healthier, and more aware. That force is quite distinct from the force that is seeking pleasure and comfort primarily.

Once in touch with the benevolent force within, ask yourself whether taking a cold shower is better for you than not taking one. If you are tapped into benevolence, that which aims to fulfill your full potential as a human being, you will know whether you are subconsciously trying to escape discomfort or there is a valid reason to skip or postpone the shower on that day.

On some days, you may feel unable to get in touch with the energy that loves you. Sometimes even when you make that conscious connection, the feeling of reluctance is not relieved. In fact, this happened to me the very morning that I wrote this sentence. I woke up not feeling very well physically. My body felt weak, delicate, even.

I meditated to clarity but still felt the reluctance. I knew that if I actually needed to, I would be able to wade into an icy river as necessary and still be aware, but considering that there was no need, for the sake of my physical health, skipping the shower felt most appropriate.

I teach TEM Daily Guided Meditations online to thousands of people each morning for 15 minutes. The class was rapidly approaching, so I decided to postpone the shower and see how the body felt after the session.

After the session was over, I sat there in a meditated state, still feeling the reluctance. I realized that I would have to find an even gentler approach if my body were going to get in the cold shower that day. My general rule is not to force my body to do things, especially if it is not feeling healthy. To do so would defy trust and could eventually lead to more bodily resistance in other areas of my life. Trust should not be betrayed.

I ran through various gradual approaches to see how my body felt toward each. Bottom up approach–no. Sink method–no. Gradual warm to cold–no.

I had never before needed an approach that was more gradual than the aforementioned options. Clearly, today my body needed something gentler still.

A moment later the image of filling up the bathtub with warm water and then starting the shower with warm water that would ever so gradually be turned to cold came to mind. The resistance disappeared.

No matter how long you have practiced, and no matter how generally healthy your body and mind are, there may still be days when the body is not feeling healthy enough to face the cold. Forcing it to do so on those days could push an already stressed immune system over the edge, leading to subsequent illness.

Rather than pushing on such days, try combining the various gradual approaches to see what your body will agree to. For example, in my case, when the right approach came to mind, my body let go of the reluctance and easily entered and enjoyed the shower. After the shower was complete, my body felt orders of magnitude better. A day when lethargy would likely lead to little if any productivity turned into a highly productive day of writing. Be creative and negotiate to find what your body will do when the normal options conjure up too much resistance. Doing so, you will likely find a way forward.

Chapter 14

The Power of One Breath

My teacher's dojo in Japan is named Ikkokukan, which translates into English as "the school of one breath." When I first began training there, I thought nothing about the name, for I was merely interested in technical training. After I matured through the training, I asked my teacher about the name.

As it turns out, he had many profound reasons for his choice of Ikkokukan. Of those, one is key to the type of training that we are encountering through this book. I would like to share that meaning with you here.

He chose the name Ikkokukan because it reminded him that life does not reside in the past or in the future, but instead in the one borrowed breath that we experience in this moment. Our physical lives end upon the final exhale. He felt the name represented the essence of the martial arts, which is revealed through vibrant present awareness.

His words reminded me of the teaching of Bushido, the code of the warrior, regarding making decisions. The basic idea is that when one makes a goal or decision, one must take some immediate positive action on that goal or decision to birth it into the world. The distance between a decision and action should not be more than one breath. If a person postpones action beyond the time it takes for a single breath, it usually means productive action will not be taken.

I began reflecting on my history of goal-making, and I realized that I had a strong record of accomplishing the aims I had set forth, so I thought I must have been doing something right. I was unwittingly following the principle of one breath in my daily life by consistently taking immediate action on my decisions, usually in the form of writing them down in a pocket notebook that I always carried with me.

What would happen was this: an inspiration would arise within me, often during my busy workday. Because I was concerned that I would not be able to recall the inspiration by the end of the day, I began carrying a pocket notebook and pen with me wherever I went.

For the most part, I was taking notes on my martial arts practice and the experiments that I wanted to perform in my martial studies. Whenever an idea came, if possible, I would immediately stop what I was doing for a moment and write a word or two that would remind me later when I checked my notebook. Later, usually when I was on the train, I would write more detail if it were necessary, so that when I read the passage the next time, I would know what I had meant.

Every now and again, I would look back over my old notebooks and see the aims and goals that were written down and be astonished at how much progress I had made. It had not occurred to me that writing only a few words might be helping to birth the goal into the world, but in retrospect, I feel that the shorthand notes did exactly that. Writing down the inspiration that arose from the subconscious seemed to align my conscious mind with the subconscious mind, priming the entire body for follow-through.

If you feel unable to immediately write something down, remember that the key to the one breath principle is that you take positive action toward the decision as soon as the decision is made. That means you could take a positive action by simply preparing to write.

For example, when I was a middle school teacher, I would often be teaching a class when something came up. If it was not possible to write it down at that moment, I would simply pull out my notebook and hold it in my hand or place it on the teacher's podium as a message to myself to write at the next available opportunity. Merely pulling the notebook out was enough to ensure that the writing would happen, and that would ensure a full follow-through later.

Of course, some people feel highly averse to writing. If that sounds like you, record your thoughts using your smart phone or a pocket recorder. The key point is to act without delay. Immediate action will rapidly weaken the habit of procrastination and lead you to a more engaging life.

You might be wondering how the one breath theory works with the type of training found in this book. As you may have experienced from your training with daily cold showers, your mind will play all sorts of games to lengthen the time between thinking of the shower and doing it. If you watch your life, you will notice that the same delay tactics come into play when you consider doing anything beneficial that strongly challenges your comfort zone.

As those healthy challenges are potentially life-transforming, finding the ability to set the goal and move toward it without delay is crucial to the potential transformation. As you repeatedly unlock inner doors with that magic key, a psychological momentum builds that will make it ever easier to take on larger and even more beneficial action thereafter.

Say, for example, you want to ask a certain person out on a date, but you are extremely nervous to do so. Thinking about it more will cause even greater anxiety. It would be better to immediately address the person with honesty, saying something like, "I feel so nervous to talk to you, but I want to get to know you better. Would you like to have a cup of tea with me after work?"

Unless the person is extremely disagreeable or narcissistic, they will at least respect your honesty because we all know how awkward asking someone out can be. Naked honesty is refreshing and will put most people at ease.

If you are on the date and you find you don't know what to say, instead of droning on in your mind about not knowing what to say, you could simply say, "I don't know what to say, but I would like to get to know you better. I wonder if you have ever felt like that before?" Everyone has felt this way at some time in their lives. By showing your feelings honestly, you have demonstrated courage while simultaneously creating the perfect opportunity for the person to open up about a time when they felt awkward, just like you. Like magic, you are getting to know each other.

All you have is one breath. In truth, you don't even have that much, because your breath is borrowed. If you are going to do anything useful in life, you are going to have to take action with that one borrowed breath. To wait any longer than one breath is to miss life.

Part V

Meditation Training

As our aim is to move toward greater and greater awareness in our daily lives, it is essential that we learn a form of meditation that blends well with our daily activities and that can stand up to the pressures of our training. Ultimately, our aim is to embody the principles of meditation, the result of which is unshakable awareness.

It is easy to assume that the challenges to meditation and awareness are merely mental and emotional, but when we begin to test our meditative abilities under pressure, we rapidly discover that the mental and emotional bottlenecks are but a small portion of the actual challenge. The fact is that a significant portion of our challenges along the meditative path relate to our physical health, specifically regarding the sympathetic nervous system. To embody meditative awareness, we need to understand the physical bottlenecks that can cause the sympathetic nervous system to switch into fight-or-flight mode. When the sympathetic nervous system is in charge, meditative awareness is furthest from our experience.

Because traditional meditation focuses on creating an ideal meditation situation, those methods rarely, if ever, challenge our physical bottlenecks. To master anything, we need to consciously make ourselves uncomfortable in our attempt to stretch beyond the range of our current capacity. To develop the capacities of the physical body, we need to take on physical challenges during meditation.

Of course, the first few times that we meditate, it makes sense to limit the challenge quite a bit because simply sitting and doing nothing while awake is challenging enough. That said, within a few sessions of beginning meditation, we need to begin increasing the challenge. If we do not, then we are missing the point of the practice.

Not progressively challenging our abilities lessens our chances of embodying meditative awareness because limiting beliefs can trap us in sedentary meditation. So long as we assume that we can't, for example, move or talk in meditation, we can never escape that limiting belief. Being overly comfortable makes us weak in every way, and so we are wise to challenge our ability to meditate in uncomfortable situations. In Part V, we are going to challenge our awareness by aiming to remain meditatively aware through discomfort, using various activities and games that will help us to embody awareness in our active daily lives.

Chapter 15

Basic TEM Meditation

After training for a few weeks to a month with daily cold showers, you are likely to discover you can make all of the primary sounds A, I, U, E, O, M and N without much difficulty. You may still have some minor lung contractions, but, more or less, you can make all the sounds reasonably.

Once you get to that point, it's time to begin a powerful meditative practice that can blend with our active daily life. Before we get to that, however, we require a basic understanding of what meditation is and how it is different from your habitual state of mind.

The brain emits several distinct brain waves that represent nervous system states. The states that we most often experience are beta, alpha, theta, and delta. Two of those states occur primarily during sleep, namely theta and delta. One state, gamma, is measured mostly in advanced meditators.

During our daily life, the brain typically inhabits two primary brainwave states. The state experienced in a given moment depends on the person's psychological condition and the activity in which the individual is partaking. For the purposes of explanation, I will explain the most focused state first because that is what people in the modern world experience most during the day. Once we have an understanding of that focused state, we will use it as our foundation to explain the other states.

If you've ever watched a cat stalking a mouse, you might notice that the cat's entire body is zeroed in on the target. During that time, the cat's attention focuses exclusively on the target. Counter to what we might assume, during its stalk, the cat, like all other predators, is most vulnerable. While stalking, predators are so completely present to that activity that they are almost entirely oblivious to all else that is happening around them. If you wait until the cat is truly committed to the stalk, so long as you are quiet, you can actually walk right up to it and touch it before it is aware you are there. Fair warning: the cat will not be very happy with you for doing this.

If you pay attention to your own life, when you are working toward an aim, you can become frustrated or annoyed when anything or anyone gets in your way. Frustration erupts because your mind has focused to exclusion, as if you were a predator stalking prey. At such times anything or anyone that interrupts us is instantly interpreted as an obstacle. If we let the initial flash of emotion express, we might say or do something inappropriate.

The brainwave state of predation is represented by the focused beta wave. Modern humans, overall, are unaware of stalking an animal, but we are very familiar with how it feels to focus our attention on a specific task to the exclusion of all else.

Beta wave helps us to focus, but it is not a healthy state to be in for long. It certainly should not be the default mode in which we live our lives. Due to our hectic lifestyles, though, beta has become the default brain wave state of our day because we are taught from early childhood to always pay attention and focus to exclusion for long periods of time.

Maintaining beta wave for too long leads to anxiety and the fight-or-flight response, also associated with a beta brain wave. When the fight-

or-flight response kicks in, it means your body is experiencing a type of anxiety that a prey creature, like a mouse, likely experiences when it catches the scent of a cat in the air. Although the anxiety that we feel is not as intense and acute as a that of a mouse who smells a cat, it is, nonetheless, taxing on the body and brain.

When we are feeling anxiety and stress, our nervous system is in prey mode, high beta wave state, which is a highly unhealthy state to sustain for long periods of time. These days, large percentages of people live in a near constant or chronic state of anxiety, which can, over time, lead to inflammatory pain, sickness, disease, and depression.

Human beings, like other hunting animals, have evolved under the pressures of predation, so we have the potential to experience both predator and prey modes. We experience the beta wave predator mode through the intense, task-oriented activities of our day, even though we may have never stalked an animal in our lives. Ironically, we also cross over into prey mode, which is also a beta wave state, when our task-oriented focus lasts too long, causing stress, or when a deadline seems to be stalking up behind us. So many of us in the modern world bounce from predator to prey mode over and over throughout our daily life—beta wave states. It's exhausting.

If we are living a balanced life, when our brains tire, we will allow ourselves to stop and rest for a time. When that happens, the brain wave switches from beta to alpha, and the body switches into parasympathetic "rest-and-digest" nervous system mode. During the rest-and-digest mode, the body is saving energy and recovering. After some recovery, we can go back to focusing on tasks for a time.

Human beings, if living a healthy life, rarely enter the anxiety-causing prey mode state. When they do enter prey mode, it is usually for a very compelling reason, and does not last for long. When our lives go out of balance, fight-or-flight anxiety can begin to creep into every moment, making us defensive and leading to withdrawal or aggressiveness for seemingly insignificant reasons.

The three states–focus, rest, and anxiety–are experienced by most people every day of their lives, at least to some degree. For most of us, those three states are all that we know. There is still another state that we can access, but that few people ever experience, which is what I call conscious alpha.

Meditative awareness allows access to a conscious alpha wave state. With a little practice with the Total Embodiment Method, we can learn to be meditatively aware through activity, which was one of the secrets of master Samurai. One of the easiest ways to begin accessing conscious alpha during activities lies in how we use our eyes and attention.

Imagine being on the battlefield surrounded by opponents aiming to kill you. If you focus your eyes and your attention like a predator, you will likely be killed by the opponents who are at your side or behind you. If you go into the defensive mode of prey species, you will be filled with anxiety and easily dispatched. To survive, you need to find another way, one that is neither predator nor prey. You may never find yourself on the battlefield surrounded by opponents, but you do experience daily conflict of the mind.

The manic nature of the mind frets over not being paid attention to, being paid too much attention, not having a job, having a job, not having enough money, having too much money, being single, being married, trouble with our children, the regret of not having children, the future, the past, et cetera. The list goes on and on. Much like on the battlefield, no matter which way we turn, there is something taking a swipe, keeping us in a state of anxiety.

The single most helpful response to those anxieties is to shift your brain into a state that is not disturbed by useless concerns, but that will take constructive action where helpful. You can't make your co-workers behave or do their jobs better. Nor can you change your boss's demeanor, but if you can shift into a conscious alpha wave state, you can take decisive action when the moment is right.

Visual Awareness Meditation

We can initially practice this meditation in a quiet room, where we will not be disturbed. Once we get a basic feel for it, which should not take more than a session or two, we can extend the practice to other environments.

Set a timer to 15 minutes so you do not have to think about time during the meditation practice. For explanation purposes, let's assume you are practicing this meditation in your bedroom.

Without taking any special pose, sit comfortably with your eyes open. Defocus your mind and gaze straight ahead with the aim of viewing the entire visual field.

To be sure you are seeing the entire visual field, without moving your eyes, make a mental note of a place on the right side, for example an object or a point on the wall that marks the outer edge of your visual field. Once you have noted that object or place, do the same thing with the left side, making note of what you can just barely see while gazing straight ahead. Finally, notice the highest and lowest points.

The general shape of our visual field is binocular. For the average person, the range of the horizontal field is about 180 degrees, while the vertical range is around 90 degrees. People with brain or eye damage may see less. If you are seeing less and were unaware that you might have a health issue related to your eyes or your brain, it is wise to consult your health practitioner. For the purposes of our meditation, however, it is only important to notice where your personal visual limits are and then be aware of the total field that you can see.

These four mental markers serve to remind you to be broadly aware without returning to the habitual focused vision. We will also keep the mind defocused. We want to guide the mind away from trying to identify objects within the visual field.

The habit of identifying can be strong for beginners, with the mind naming everything that catches your attention–"TV," "clock", "chipped paint," et cetera. Every time your mind makes an identification, relax a bit more and return to total visual awareness. Practicing in this way over a period of weeks, the mind quickly releases the tendency to focus and identify, at least while you are meditating.

If you can remain aware of the total visual field and relax, your brain will soon emit a conscious alpha wave, which indicates you are in a state of meditation. When in conscious alpha, your body and brain will be conserving energy and recovering from the stress that the habitual task-oriented, anxiety stimulating beta wave state has created.

The goal with your initial practice is to remain in a relaxed awareness of the entire visual field for 15 minutes. If you notice your mind keeps trying to focus or if it wanders, just relax and return awareness to the content of the total visual field. Be careful not to bulge the eyes, however, for doing so will likely result in neck and shoulder tension and possibly a headache. Along with relaxing the eyes, be sure to relax the lips, jaw, neck, shoulders, hands, and your breathing.

You may be surprised to discover that the total visual field you are now seeing is the field your eyes pick up at all times but your brain selectively blocks from your accessible memory. Usually your visual awareness is limited primarily to that which your brain finds interesting.

After 15 minutes of seated visual awareness meditation, it's time to start challenging yourself a bit. You might first try to look around with defocused eyes. You could then try moving an arm or a leg. If you are able to remain peripherally aware, try getting up and sitting down again. Try walking around. Through all these activities, keep the mind and the eyes defocused.

Before long, you will realize you can remain meditated and move freely. In initial practice sessions, you will probably look and feel a bit awkward. Maybe you represent the zombie apocalypse that so many people fear at the end of days! Jokes aside, with practice, you will soon be able to walk normally when peripherally aware—a stealth zombie, if you will.

As we are practicing a visual meditation that depends on peripheral vision, let's take note of the differences between foveal (focused) and peripheral (defocused) vision. You might note that foveal vision is high definition color-rich vision, while peripheral vision is much lower in definition and color deficient.

Most importantly, bring your awareness to the feeling that foveal vision creates in the body as compared to that of peripheral vision. Foveal vision creates physical tension, whereas peripheral vision relaxes the body. If you felt that change, it means you noticed the difference between beta and alpha brain waves!

The advantages of focused vision are you can see more color and detail than you can when using peripheral vision. The disadvantage of foveal vision, aside from the tension it creates, is that it is insensitive to movement and leads to an almost complete lack of awareness of what occurs just outside the line of focus.

To get an impactful experience of how foveal vision works, type "Test of Selective Attention" in your web browser and enjoy the video. Spoiler alert: reading beyond this point without watching the video will spoil the video experience.

I hope you enjoyed that video. If you didn't get it right the first time, do not be concerned, for the vast majority of people miss it. In any case, the experiment reflects how blind the brain is to information in the immediate environment when we are using foveal vision.

Another example of the blindness of foveal vision occurs when you read. As you read, notice how you are almost entirely unaware of what occurs beyond the page unless you make a concerted effort to see what's happening beyond the text. You might also observe that when you make a concerted effort to extend awareness beyond the page, you are unable to read. Or if you can actually sound out the words, you are much less able to comprehend and remember the content than you would be if you focused on reading alone. With practice, you will eventually be able to read, fully comprehend, and see the entire room naturally.

Although peripheral vision is color-deficient and lacking in detail, it leads to an awareness of our environment and is much more sensitive to movement and shades than is color-rich foveal vision. These advantages reflect the hemisphere of the brain through which they are being processed. For most right-handed people, focused vision is processed by the left hemisphere, which is primarily dedicated to identity and thought, whereas peripheral vision is processed in the right hemisphere, which is primarily dedicated to feeling, emotion and awareness. For left-handed people, the hemispheres are reversed.

Returning to the meditation, it's important to remember that persistence is essential to quality of life improvement. With an active daily meditation practice, you will discover that the stimuli which used to easily pull you out of conscious alpha have lost their impact on you. Still other challenges will have lessened their distractive allure for you. These are great signs of progress.

Meditating Under Pressure

Note: for safety, always set a timer for 10 minutes to remind you to get out before hypothermia sets in.

Within a few days of practicing conscious alpha through the visual awareness meditation, begin to challenge your meditative abilities in the cold shower. To do so, prior to entering the bathroom, get yourself into a meditated state via the visual awareness meditation.

Maintain defocused vision and mind while moving and taking off your clothing. Relax the body and mind deeply without thinking about the shower. If you can, get in the shower without a single thought of the cold water. Be sure you are still meditated before starting the shower. See if you can turn on the water while maintaining physical and mental relaxation. Keep the eyes unfocused.

If you find your mind or body tenses with anticipation when you look at the shower knob, then you know it is the fear and anticipation of discomfort that has pulled you out of primary awareness. At this stage, simply notice what the mind does. There is nothing special you need to do about the tension other than to relax the body and defocus the mind again while gazing at the shower knob.

Once relaxed, begin your shower by directing the cold water flow to your feet via the gradual approach that we learned in Chapter 8. Whenever you feel your meditation break or weaken, redirect the shower head away and get back into the meditation before returning to the gradual process. Go as far as you can while remaining meditated.

The real challenge will be when the showerhead is spraying cold water into your face, for at that time, you will have to close your eyes. The temptation will be to focus the mind on the place that is being most stimulated by the water, the place that is most uncomfortable. Focusing on that area will take you out of meditation in an instant. Remember to relax as much as possible and remain mentally defocused.

Generally speaking, once a person can make all the sounds in the cold shower, they can usually complete a full cold shower in meditative awareness. If you are not quite at the place where you can remain in meditation through a full cold shower, do not be concerned, for it is not a race. With a little more practice, you will get there.

Whether or not you maintained the meditation perfectly while in the shower, be sure you are in conscious alpha (meditative awareness) when you exit the shower. Dry yourself and get dressed while in meditation. Exit the bathroom and see how long you can go through your daily activities while aware.

Chapter 16

Spherical Awareness

Awareness was one of the most essential qualities of a master Samurai. He used each moment of his life as an opportunity to train awareness, so that it would be there at all times. His aim was for awareness to be his eyes, his hands, his feet, his sword and his shield, his heart. He wasn't satisfied until awareness was there while eating, while urinating, in conversation, in his sleep, during sex—in every moment.

Achieving such a degree of awareness sounds like hard work. If trained properly, it is certainly challenging, but there is never a dull moment. Once you get the hang of the training, you'll notice things you've never noticed before. A whole new world of exploration and adventure opens for you. Each moment offers a chance for living more fully.

Spherical Awareness Meditation

Imagine you are walking alone down a dark alley late at night, something I hope you never do. Now imagine you hear footsteps behind you as you walk. Quite naturally, your mind is going to be highly attentive to the space behind you as you walk, even if you are looking forward.

As you walk further, the footsteps seem to be a little louder, seeming to be closer. Your heartbeat elevates, and you start feeling anxiety. Your mind starts conjuring images of the thug behind you, of being mugged, raped, or otherwise assaulted.

The first feeling you are likely to experience is an inner war between wanting to turn around and look and the incredible fear of doing exactly that. The fear suggests that turning around will instigate an attack. Most feel deep anxiety as their nervous system goes into fight-or-flight mode. This response makes sense absent a better strategy. Fight-or-flight is a panic response that blocks awareness. Fortunately, there is another way, spherical awareness.

The key to spherical awareness is found in the scenario above, specifically the ability to be sensitive to the area behind you even though your eyes are looking forward. During that situation, your mind is doing something especially important, in that it is intentionally feeling behind you even though technically speaking your physical senses are weak or inoperable in that direction.

Despite the sensory blind spot, you are being attentive in that direction. In truth, you can be attentive in any direction in a similar fashion. It's easiest to notice this capacity, at first, when you imagine that someone is out to get you. Try it and see for yourself. While looking straight ahead, briefly flash your attention to your left side without physically looking there. Now do the same thing with your right side. Try it again while being attentive behind you. Do it one more time in each direction rapidly, left, right, behind, up, and down. Now try it again but with relaxation. How does that feel?

What if, through relaxation, you could be attentive in every direction simultaneously? How would that feel? You can. Try it and see for yourself. What does it feel like?

Many of my students report that after they consciously develop this sense, it feels as if something has opened up within them. That's exactly how I feel it too. I wonder if you can feel that opening. If not, with time it will come. Once you experience it, you will understand what I mean. You won't be able to explain this change to anyone in a way that they will understand until they too have experienced the shift.

So, what is the difference between the anxious awareness of the person who was being followed and what you are doing now? Primarily, the difference is in the state of the nervous system. In the stalking scenario, you are likely in a highly anxious, fearful state, a sympathetic nervous system response known as fight-or-flight. When in that state, the nervous system is behaving very similarly to how a mouse feels when it detects the smell of a cat in the air. The feeling is small and reactive.

When in fight-or-flight, an individual is likely to panic, which will result in one of three scenarios. The most common is avoidance, when the mind tries to talk itself out of the belief that there is danger: "I'm imagining things," or "He's not stalking me; he just happens to be heading in the same direction as I am." Those justifications may or may not be reflective of reality. If there were a real stalker behind you, avoidance puts you in a highly vulnerable position indeed.

The second scenario, also a fight-or-flight response, is to break into a panicked run, which will likely spur the stalker, if there is one, to chase you, much like a cat instinctively chases a ball. If you are a fast runner, you may escape. However, because of panic, you will likely experience an adrenaline dump, which means your body will quickly exhaust itself. If the stalker is in decent shape, they will likely catch you, and if they do, you may be so tired you can no longer effectively think or do anything useful.

In the third scenario, one might be in the fight aspect of fight-or-flight, deciding to turn and attack whoever is behind you. Because you are responding in a kind of panicked state like an animal that has been backed into a corner, again you suffer the adrenaline dump and exhaust quickly. If you are lucky, the stalker, assuming there is a stalker, will be caught off guard and overwhelmed. If they have a weapon, you will likely be injured or killed.

All three of those reactions have nothing to do with meditation or awareness as I mean the term. For there to be awareness, as I use the term, we must not be caught in the extreme beta wave, sympathetic nervous response of fight-or-flight but instead in the conscious alpha wave state of spherical awareness, like that of a master Samurai surrounded by opponents intent on cutting him down. Even with death staring him down, he is calm, centered, and aware in every direction, trusting that his aware body will reveal the best path through the encounter.

When in fight-or-flight mode, undue tension builds up in your body, making your movements stiff. Your attention is focused in one direction, and you present an energy of weakness. That picture draws attention of would-be attackers, much like an injured elk draws the eyes of the wolf pack. Simply being unaware draws the attention of would-be attackers because the body language reflects vulnerability.

When one remains in a centered spherical awareness, predators feel deterred because limiting risk is an instinctive priority for them. There is no need to puff up and try to look tough, for that is not awareness, and is as likely to result in a violent confrontation.

Instead of trying to look tough, remain calm and centered. This quality of energy has an amazing effect on would-be predators. Most of them are confused by a calm and aware demeanor. Confusion when under pressure creates fear. Suddenly, the predator is uncertain, and that uncertainty tends to result in withdrawal.

As a young man, I was unexpectedly able to test out calm, centered awareness under the threat of muggers on several occasions, each resulting in apparent confusion on the part of the muggers and a peaceful withdrawal. My rushed state of mind attracted their attention.

Once they began their approach, I noticed them and the energy that I was projecting that had caught their attention. In that instant, I became spherically aware. They backed off without any need for aggressive words or a violent confrontation. At first, I was confused by their odd responses to my calm awareness, but after training for a sufficient period of time and testing the power of spherical awareness over and over, I realized that people in predator mode are confused by this state of being.

The nervous systems of all animals, humans included, have evolved over the eons to sense four nervous system states. The first state is that of a lack of awareness or inattentiveness, the easiest target. The second state is that of avoidance or denial, another easy target. You can see this state in animals, who when nervous look away from the stressor, but do not run away. The third state is flight, which results in a chase, making it much more challenging than inattentiveness or avoidance. The fourth state is that of aggression, where an animal will turn and fight the attacker.

Most encounters in nature result in chases because animals generally enter into flight mode more easily than they do avoidance, and of course wild animals are a lot more attentive than humans are because they must be to survive. Of the four states, the most challenging is when an animal turns and fights. Most predators are not prepared for that. The typical result of a fight is injury to both parties, so aiming for an animal that is likely to turn and fight is a poor strategy for a lone predator. Most predators will try to avoid animals that they feel will go into fight mode unless the predators greatly outnumber the prey.

There is another state, however, to which the default nervous system seems completely blind—calm spherical awareness. Animals seem incapable of choosing this state, but humans, if made aware of it, can. With practice, humans can begin to embody this type of awareness throughout their daily life.

Pressure-Training Spherical Awareness

Note: for safety, always set a timer for 10 minutes to remind you to get out before hypothermia sets in.

Now that you are familiar with spherical awareness, it is important you begin putting it into practice and developing it through progressive challenges. We can use the cold shower to begin pressure-training spherical awareness.

Get into a calm spherical awareness prior to entering the bathroom. Once calm and aware, enter, disrobe, and step into the shower while remaining spherically aware.

Once in the shower, gaze at the shower knob and then the shower head to see if anticipation pulls you out of awareness. To test your awareness in this way simply place the shower knob or shower head in the center of your visual awareness without focusing on them. If you can keep your mind from focusing, you should be able to remain spherically aware.

Turn on the shower with the aim of maintaining this state throughout the watery chaos. Keep a light awareness on the space around you, such that if someone were to enter the room, you would calmly notice.

Once the shower is complete, exit and dry yourself while maintaining spherical awareness. Get dressed and see how long you can maintain it through the rest of your day.

A person who is not quite ready for the spherical awareness pressure challenge may notice that their energy collapses back to smallness at the thought of the shower or when the cold hits the skin. They may even notice that their attention moves inward defensively because bodily systems are not yet strong enough to remain aware under pressure. Even individuals who have meditated for many years will be unable to meditate in a cold shower if they have not trained their bodies properly.

The bottom line is that weak-energy individuals are unable to meditate unless they are comfortable. As we are training ourselves to be unshakably aware, the unconscious dependence on comfort must be overcome, because life is often uncomfortable. If the practitioner does not transcend the comfort barrier, there will be a continual separation between meditative awareness and daily life. Therefore, only by challenging meditative abilities through discomfort will we fully embody awareness in our lives.

Chapter 17

Deeper Bodily Training

The most challenging time for the cold shower is 3 to 4 AM, when the body's blood pressure and hormonal activity are at the lowest point. You might notice that when you are sick the symptoms always feel worst around this time. Those early morning hours are also when the majority of people die in their sleep. Of course, if you get up at 5 or 6 AM and head straight into the shower, your blood pressure will likely be higher than at 3 AM, but it would still be quite low compared to other times of your waking day, so taking your cold shower in the morning is a solid challenge. By contrast, the easiest time to take a cold shower is when you are fully awake and your blood pressure is up to normal. If you have been conducting your cold shower training during those relatively easy times, then you might be tempted to think you have mastered the method when you have not.

The way to mastery is to take showers in the early morning when the body is still relatively low on energy. If you can take those showers in seamless spherical awareness, then you know you are ready for the next step, which we will explore in this chapter.

Once we have mastered the shower through spherical awareness, that means we are no longer hesitant to enter the shower unless we are feeling ill. New challenges still lie before us if we wish, for example, such as taking cold baths.

Before partaking in that type of training, be sure to consult your health practitioner. If you have a heart condition or Raynaud's Syndrome, it may be best to avoid cold baths altogether until you have successfully overcome those conditions. If you never intend to take a cold bath, you might skip from here to the next chapter to resume your progress without cold baths.

Before we get into the specific methods and reasons for taking a cold bath, let's begin with exceptions: when an otherwise healthy person who had decided to partake in cold baths might want to skip them on certain days.

Sick Days

If you are not feeling well one morning, you might omit the cold bath and even the cold shower and instead use only the sink method described in chapter 8. If your energy is extremely low, you have a fever, chills, or signs of sickness, avoid all forms of cold training as they can weaken your body even further. Take a rest on days like that.

If you are not feeling sick, but feel a bit low on energy, you might continue your training via the sink method detailed in Chapter 8.

I began my cold water training in a creek during survival training. It was so humid during the summer that I found I could not sleep at night. I began wading into the creek at night with the intention of cooling down my body just so I could get a good night's sleep. It worked extremely well.

Once I returned to Tokyo, also a humid place, I continued doing the same thing but with cold baths. We lived in an apartment that did not have a cooling system, so nights were sweaty and uncomfortable. The cold baths greatly enhanced my sleep quality.

From that training, I stopped wearing heavy clothing in the winter, such that my clothing selection between summer and winter varied little. To this day, I enjoy cold baths more than I do cold showers. As I indicated earlier, Raynaud's Syndrome seems to run in my family, so I need to be mindful about taking cold baths and wearing more clothing during the cold seasons.

Cold water immersions present different challenges than cold showers. Baths are not as chaotic as the showers, but they are more physically challenging than cold showers. Cold baths challenge composure because they remove the heat from your body more quickly than cold showers do, but quietly.

Assuming you are fit to take a cold bath, as judged by you and your health practitioner, it is important you first know the symptoms of hypothermia. A failure to recognize the symptoms can lead to death.

Symptoms of Hypothermia

According to the Mayo Clinic, the signs of hypothermia are as follows:

- Shivering
- Slurred speech or mumbling
- Slow, shallow breathing
- Weak pulse
- Clumsiness or lack of coordination
- Drowsiness or extremely low energy
- Confusion or memory loss
- Loss of consciousness

As the Mayo Clinic warns, "Someone with hypothermia usually isn't aware of his or her condition because the symptoms often begin gradually." The website also notes that "confused thinking associated with hypothermia prevents self-awareness," which can "lead to risk-taking behavior."

The Mayo Clinic further lists a number of risk factors that can increase the odds of getting hypothermia (see "Hypothermia" on Mayo Clinic website):

- Fatigue or exhaustion will reduce your tolerance for cold.
- Older age can reduce the body's ability to regulate body temperature and to sense the symptoms of hypothermia.
- In adolescence the body loses heat faster than is common with adults.
- Mental problems such as dementia and other conditions may interfere with judgment or awareness of the symptoms of hypothermia as they set in.
- Alcohol causes the blood vessels to expand, which can make the body feel warm. Due to the expansion of the blood vessels when they should be contracting to protect from the cold, the body will lose heat more rapidly. Furthermore, alcohol diminishes the natural shivering response, which is one of the first signs you need to get out of the water. With alcohol, there is also a risk of passing out in the water.
- Recreational drugs affect judgment and can lead to passing out in the cold water.
- Medical conditions that affect regulation of body temperature such as hypothyroidism, anorexia nervosa, diabetes, stroke, severe arthritis, Parkinson's disease, trauma, and spinal cord injuries increase the risk of hypothermia.
- Medications such as antidepressants, antipsychotics, pain medications, and sedatives can reduce the body's ability to regulate heat.

The takeaway is simple: cold bath training should be done by individuals who are ready to take their training seriously and have consulted their health practitioner. If you notice any of the symptoms of hypothermia, cease the exposure immediately and warm your body.

As a general rule, do not stay in the cold water for more than 10 minutes. Once your body has become highly conditioned to cold and you have become extremely familiar with the signs of hypothermia, you might be able to stay in longer.

Cold Bath Meditation

Note: for safety, always set a timer for 10 minutes to remind you to get out before hypothermia sets in.

Once your circulatory system and cells have become strong and vibrantly healthy, taking cold baths will allow you to enjoy a powerful and blissful meditation.

Here is how to take a basic meditative cold bath:

- Be sure you are in spherical awareness prior to entering the cold bath.
- See if you can step in and sit down in one seamless, aware, harmonious motion that flows into the next movement, without pause or haste.
- Once seated, slowly extend your legs to immerse them fully in the water.
- Once your legs are fully wet, hold your breath and lie back as gracefully as possible to submerge your torso and head.
- Remain submerged for as long as you can comfortably hold your breath, while in spherical awareness.
- Once you are ready to take your next breath, sit up and fully relax in a deep meditation.
- As you sit there, your body heat will warm the water near it, and that will create an insulative barrier from the coldest water. Every now and again use your hands and legs to gracefully move

the water around so your body experiences the coldest temperatures available.

- After a minute or so of sitting in meditation, with grace, hold your breath and re-submerge your upper body and head until you are ready to take another breath.
- At the ten-minute mark (or before if you are experiencing any symptoms of hypothermia), exit the bathtub gracefully in spherical awareness.
- Dry off and get dressed and continue your day in spherical awareness.

Once you get the hang of remaining spherically aware through the basic bath that I outlined above, forget the form, and do whatever feels right while you are in the cold bath, while being mindful of safety precautions. Feel your way through the experience from a deep spherical awareness.

Chapter 18

Awareness Exercises and Games

To discover unshakable awareness, it is vital to begin integrating spherical awareness into daily life both within and outside the house. We want awareness to penetrate all the way down to and affect us at the level of instinct.

For human beings, the same as with animals, game play is a powerful way to get in touch with instinct. If you were a hunter-gatherer, no matter where you lived around the world, you would be likely to encounter some variant of the exercises and games included in this chapter.

In my personal pursuit of incorporating awareness, I made up a number of these exercises and games, only later to discover that people have been doing them for ages. The tools found in this chapter will add a little spice to your daily practice and serve to keep you aware when you might otherwise not be. I hope you enjoy them as much as I do.

X-Ray Vision

The first exercise is pretending you have X-Ray Vision. You may have imagined you had X-Ray Vision when you were a child. This game differs from the one you likely played then. The basis of this exercise is spherical awareness, which we will combine with an imaginary map that we constantly update as we practice.

With open eyes, imagine you had X-Ray Vision that allowed you to see through walls to the rooms, doors, hallways, et cetera, that lay beyond your physical sight. If you are outdoors, you could visualize the lay of the land, the trees, hills, rivers, et cetera, that are beyond your physical sight. Create a low detail 3-D mental map of your surroundings such that if you closed your eyes, you could imagine the entire space that includes the obvious objects like furniture (there is no need to go high definition with your imagination by trying to visualize the texture of the walls or the strokes in a painting).

This exercise will keep you paying attention to the area around you, and that attentiveness will allow you to keep the mental map relatively up to date. As you practice this exercise, you will be more motivated to travel about so you can discover what lies beyond your physical awareness. The new information will be internally mapped and included in your X-Ray Vision. The map will never be entirely correct, but it will help you to practice spherical awareness while at the same time keep you physically paying attention to the space around you.

Spinning with X-Ray Vision

This is an extension of the X-Ray Vision exercise.

1. Stand up and look around you to create a mental map of your surroundings.

2. Once you have your surroundings mapped, extend your awareness over the entire area spherically as you have already learned to do.
3. Once awareness is extended, close your eyes while activating your imaginary X-Ray Vision and begin to turn slowly in place like the hand of a clock.
4. While slowly turning with eyes closed, select an object like a room or a door to point out after you have taken several 360-degree rotations.
5. As soon as you feel that room or object is lined up with your nose, stop and point to it with your eyes still closed.
6. Open your eyes to check your accuracy.

Playing this game often will develop an incredibly powerful map of your surroundings at all times, while simultaneously training spherical awareness.

Topographical View

Topography is the study of the features and shape of the land. Topographical viewing is an exercise that most hunter-gatherers practice so that they do not get lost. As they walk along, they imagine that their spirit is high above their body looking down to see the lay of the land, its prominent features and shapes.

The imaginary view would include mountains, valleys, rivers, creeks, forests, meadows, and so on. If you were in the city, it would include buildings, streets, corners, business sectors and neighborhoods, highlands and lowlands.

From a meditated state, imagine that your "spiritual eye" rises out of your body, moving high into the air to look down upon the topography surrounding you. As you move around, keep updating the topographical view.

Many people who practice this exercise find that they feel pleasantly high while doing it. The feeling results from a shift to a conscious brain wave state. If you play this game as you walk, it becomes increasingly less likely you will get lost.

Assassin Game

This is an excellent awareness game that at once stimulates instinct and spherical awareness. The idea is to expand your awareness through the entire space of your home, for example, with the aim of sensing where other people are at all times. In this game, imagine other people are assassins out to get you.

To score a point, you need to notice someone approaching you before they come within 10 feet of you. If you notice them before they are within 10 feet of you, then you survived the assassin's attack. In your mind, you might tally a point. If someone approaches within 10 feet of you before you notice them, then you have been assassinated. In that case, give yourself a minus point.

There is no need to tell anyone about this game. It doesn't matter if they intend to sneak up on you or even if they were oblivious to your presence; if they come within 10 feet of you, it means you were assassinated. At the end of each day, tally up how many times you avoided the assassination as compared to how many times you were assassinated. I used to keep track of my daily tallies in my pocket notebook to help me see if there was progress over time. You might enjoy doing that as well.

As your awareness improves through this game, you will want to increase the challenges. You can easily do this by increasing the distance measurement from 10 feet to maybe 15 or 20 feet, or more as you gain ability.

Training in this way will give you the sort of sixth sense martial arts legends are said to have had. Most importantly, it stimulates instinct and awareness simultaneously, modifying your instinctive response so that it is connected to awareness in greater duration, and as that connection strengthens, you will tend to experience less anxiety about the chaos of life.

Blind Spots

Most automobile accidents occur in areas that the drivers involved are highly familiar with—like their neighborhoods. Accident statistics suggest that the closer you get to home or any road you frequently travel, the more you tend to drive on autopilot, a time when you are least aware.

Think of the number of times when you arrived at your destination unable to remember how you got there. When we repeatedly drive in highly familiar areas, we tend to rely on muscle memory and zone out. In that scenario, it makes sense that our risk of having an accident will increase.

Not only are accidents most common when we are near home, they also are more deadly because people will neglect to put their seatbelts on, or they will take them off early when they are just around the corner from home.

If you pay attention to how you drive, you will notice you are most vigilant when in unfamiliar territory. This heightened vigilance is true of most people whenever they are in a new situation, not only while driving.

If you were to watch people in a crowded city, you'd probably find it relatively easy to differentiate the tourists from the locals. Locals tend to be in a rush. They move directly from point A to point B, usually not bothering to look around—oftentimes watching their feet as they shuffle along. Tourists, on the other hand, tend to look around a lot more than the locals, which makes their path less direct and less rushed on average.

If you were an assassin making your plan, who would you like to target, the aware or the unaware individual? The unaware individual would be the safer target. To maximize your chances of success, you'd aim to meet your target at a location where they will be less alert, of course.

Most people, when they imagine a ninja assassin from ancient Japan, think of a powerfully skilled and agile young warrior in a black suit. That's Hollywood. There were skilled warriors among ninja, but most assassins and spies were women. Imagine, rather, the maid or the mistress. Lulled by a seemingly harmless image, the target usually died in their own bed or in the latrine. When we are in such places, we tend to assume that we are safe, so we allow ourselves to be fully self-absorbed.

Muggers, likewise, usually look for people who are alone and not paying attention. Counter to what people often assume, many muggings happen in broad daylight. If you were an experienced mugger, whom would you target?

When I was a young man, someone attempted to mug me in broad daylight at a bus station. I was in a rush and not paying attention. I must have looked like a perfect victim. The mugger was able to walk right up to my side and brandish a knife, nearly touching my right ribcage before I came out of my hasty stupor. Calm, spherical awareness confused him, and I was able to direct him out of his nefarious course of action. Had I remained in beta brain wave, the outcome would certainly have been different. Self-absorption is dangerous.

If you pay attention to where you look when you drive to and from work, you will notice your eyes tend to notice and miss the same things almost every drive. The same is true when you are at home walking through your house. Certain areas especially seem to catch your attention, and others you almost never notice. Those blind spots are where the assassin might be.

To get a better idea of how to repattern your awareness to notice the blind spots, start noticing where you look as you walk around your home. You will likely find you look at the same things repeatedly and consistently fail to notice other places. Simply by watching your life pattern, a skilled assassin will know what you pay attention to better than you do. To succeed in their nefarious plan, all they need to do is be in one of your blind spots as you pass.

Once you start to notice your own blind spots, start to observe the blind spots of your family members and your neighbors. Take note of their regular patterns as well. What time do they go out to get the mail, take out the garbage, leave for work, return, et cetera? Some of these areas may vary a bit, while others are extremely consistent. Persistent patterns indicate potential blind spots your imaginary assassin could use to their advantage.

The key with this game and every game is that it is practiced from a conscious alpha wave state, not beta. If you practice noticing blind spots and imagining your vulnerabilities from beta wave state, that may cause you anxiety, which would run counter to your aims. Be sure you are in an aware state with each game. And be sure to have fun with it!

Gateway Awareness

If you ever enter a restaurant or café, it would be nice to have some exercises you could play there as well. Gateway Awareness is an exercise that I learned from the teachings of Sokaku Takeda, the famous headmaster of Daito-ryu Aikijujutsu from the 20th century. Daito-ryu is a Samurai martial system that I received from Osaki Sensei while in Japan. Sokaku Takeda taught his close students that whenever entering or exiting through a gate or doorway with someone else, do what you can to be last.

The reason he gave for this practice was that, in the previous generations, many Samurai were assassinated unexpectedly by the polite person who "kindly" entered or exited behind them. The finishing method was usually a choke, garrote, or dagger drawn across the throat at the precise moment when the victim was going through the door frame or gateway, a moment when evasive movement was most limited.

Takeda Sensei was born in the era of the Samurai, and his training was severe. As a young boy, he would sneak away from home to walk onto active battlefields. He wanted to learn about the nature of war. He discovered that because he was a boy, the warriors on either side ignored him, which gave him, in his eyes, a safe education. While he was a young adult, Japan transitioned into a modern country. Samurai lost their position in society, and carrying a sword, the symbol of their feudal power, became illegal.

With a unified, modern nation, Japan became an extremely safe place to live, so warriors from the old days began to soften their safety protocols, but not Takeda Sensei. To the day he died in his eighties, he stubbornly refused to enter a building before someone else.

Of course, in our modern world, it is highly unlikely you would ever encounter an assassin, but for our purposes, warding off assassination attempts is not the point. Rather, the purpose of this game is to remind you to be spherically aware and in the best possible position every time you move through a doorway or other narrow passage.

From the perspective of those with you, your opening the door for them may be viewed as chivalrous, which is true, but being polite is not the primary reason for going in last. For training purposes, we can use all doorways, hallways, or other such narrow spaces, including the ones at home, as triggers to remind us to be spherically aware.

Each time you remember and practice spherical awareness and strategic positioning, you are restructuring your brain through neuroplasticity to access spherical awareness more easily. Let's make doorways and passages a part of your grand awareness game!

Remember, so long as our society is still relatively safe, it's a game. There is no need to get uptight about who goes last. Instead, see how often you are able to gently guide people to go before you. Have fun with it!

Seat Positioning

You have learned to successfully ward off an assassination attempt by chivalrously entering and exiting last. Now that you are through the threshold, use spherical awareness to note the general layout of the building and the exits. Notice which table provides the safest place to sit and observe. Try to choose a table that has the fewest vectors of attack while simultaneously providing for best view of the entire space.

With the criteria of safety from assassination in mind, sitting next to a window, door, or passageway, is generally ill-advised. A table in the middle of the room surrounded by other tables is also best avoided. Generally speaking, a table in a corner provides the best possible vantage point without exposing your back. If the ideal table is unavailable, aim for the next best table that provides a good view and relatively few vectors of attack.

Once you have found the best possible table, see if you can guide your group to sit there. This too is a game that will exercise your ability to lead people to safety without them necessarily recognizing the service.

To get people to sit at your selected table, you could just explain that you are learning personal defense and that selecting the safest table is part of the training. If you don't want to divulge that information, you might try framing the table in a way that seems advantageous to them. If, for example, you are on a date, you could confide with your partner that you would like that certain table because it feels more intimate. Personally, I prefer to tell the truth because it saves me a lot of time with people. If someone doesn't like the real me, then the truth has saved us both a lot of time.

After moving to the selected table, you will want to sit in the most advantageous seat for your imaginary duties as a protector. That seat will allow optimal visual awareness of the entire space, while also allowing optimal movement.

The next consideration is seating position. Sitting in the back corner of a table would be a bad idea because it will greatly limit your ability to take action, which means you are unable to protect others or escape if necessary. With freedom of movement and protective service in mind, you will want to sit with your back to a wall, if possible, but at the open end of the booth, so you could easily stand, if necessary.

Alternative Exits

Another teaching of Sokaku Takeda that makes for a great game is that of finding alternative exits. Whenever you enter a building, see if you can discover an alternative way of escaping via a back door or window. To do so, you will want to mentally map out the inner space of the building.

For example, if you were in a restaurant, once you get your party seated, you can take a few minutes to use the restroom. In spherical awareness, get up and head for the restroom while mentally mapping the layout of the place. Make note of any openable windows and doors. Glance into the kitchen to note if there is a back door. Check the bathroom for a possible window you could use as an exit.

When you become skilled at this game, it does not take long to find alternative exits. The practice saved me and a few friends from a gang when we were in high school. In the event of civil unrest, this skill can save your life. Until then, it's only a game, so have fun with it.

Part VI

Living Awareness

Traditional meditation, as it has been practiced throughout the ages, has almost without exception existed as a retreat from daily life. We are now entering a time where that separation will no longer suffice. Human beings are ready for the next evolution in consciousness, which is living awareness.

We have been conditioned to believe that meditation must be difficult and that only a very few special individuals can take that evolutionary step. To understand the falsity of this idea, let us employ a parable. Like an adult elephant at a zoo, tied by a rope which it could easily break, if only its mind was not imprisoned by a false belief, you too may come to see you can easily break formerly limiting beliefs.

So long as you believe that meditation is difficult, you are tied. The elephant came to that belief during its youth, when it was not so strong. At that developmental state, it was tied with a thick metal chain. It struggled and struggled against the chain until it eventually exhausted all will to struggle. The size of the chain was then reduced. If there was no subsequent struggle, then it was changed to a rope that it would never challenge due to the limiting belief. As an adult, the elephant could easily break a zoo rope but never tries because it believes the rope to be unbreakable.

Because traditional meditation forms require tremendous concentration to be effective, many of us believe without doubt that we can't live our lives in meditative awareness. Such a belief is reasonable, because if you have to concentrate on one thing to exclusion, you would be unable able to read, write, talk or perform any other of the many daily life functions that require a degree of focus to execute. Maybe you, like that elephant, can break that chain. You are ready to take the evolutionary step into living awareness. You may simply need a little coaching, a little direction as to how to go about taking that step.

Living through awareness will not require great will power or effort, but don't fool yourself; it will take persistence. The type of persistence is like that of a toddler learning to walk. It falls again and again, and just keeps getting up. It learns to walk not because it sets a goal and wills it to happen like an athlete or entrepreneur does. The toddler keeps trying persistently through the natural forces of curiosity and instinct. Similarly, your next steps must come of curiosity and instinct. With TEM, your largest barrier to practice will not be a lack of willpower but simply forgetting to meditate during the day. If you can remember to meditate, the process is relatively simple.

In Part VI, we are going to learn how to strategically set up awareness reminders, so you are less likely to forget about your training as you go about your active daily life. From there, you will receive a guideline to help you embody awareness each day, that incorporates the tools that this book has presented. Next, we will unveil the true nature of the force within that has been holding you back, so you can quell the war within. Finally, we will explore the nature of awareness and how personal transformation emerges as you progress along the way.

Chapter 19

Daily Reminders

One of the greatest challenges to integrating awareness in daily life is the habit of being unaware. Unless we remember to be aware, the habitual pattern will control our daily life. A true personal transformation cannot emerge when unconsciousness is the captain of your life.

I often ask students if they can quantify the percentage of their average day that they are spherically aware. Most students, the first time that I ask this question, answer between 10 and 20%. If I ask the same student that same question three to six months later, the percentage invariably goes down, not up.

Hearing that answer, we might be discouraged. Although their assessment has gone down as a result of the practice, it has done so because they come to see how unaware they are during the day, which is an improvement. The first time that I asked the question, students assumed that they were much more aware than they were in actual practice, so their estimate was generously high.

A simple way to understand the phenomenon is to reflect on what happens when the mind wanders during meditation. When the mind wanders, the individual is not lucid: at that time, they themselves do not realize that their mind has wandered. Only when lucidity returns, does the individual wake up from the unconscious daydream and notice that they were not aware. They may have a hard time quantifying how long they were unaware, but at least they know that they were unaware for a time.

Similarly, as we become more lucid in our daily lives, we are more likely to take note of the gaps of time when we were unaware. Again, such an observation only occurs after awareness returns, but at least, at that time, a mental note is taken that there was a loss of lucidity.

When I first posed the question, they had no real way to answer it because they had not been noticing when they were unaware. By the time I ask again, students have had plenty of experience noticing the loss of lucidity. From the many months of tracking gaps in awareness, they recognize that they are far less aware than they had previously assumed.

Similarly, most people who do not pay attention to their lucidity, or lack thereof, assume they are in control of their lives. Often, it is not until they start tracking their lack of awareness that they come to see that they are largely not in control of their lives. Upon taking an accounting of lucidity, they realize that they have been almost entirely stuck in a compulsive dream of the past and future—a dream of their identity.

You may wonder what I mean by a dream of identity. If you have reached a place of expanded, relaxed clarity, you will notice that during that lucidity, you have only awareness of the moment. With awareness, there is no thought about who one is, where one comes from, one's ethnicity, culture, ideology, beliefs, et cetera. There is only the awareness of whatever is happening in the instant—so the mind, and therefore identity, is quiet. By contrast, the dream of identity carries the mind away in compulsive thinking about the past and future. In any case, there is little or no control when we are trapped in the dream of identity.

The key to inner freedom is to remember to practice awareness during your day. The question is, when we are stuck in the dream of time, as we almost always are, how do we remember to practice awareness? That's what the content of this chapter is here to show you.

If you incorporate the tools of this chapter into your daily life, you will remember more often and that will help to break you out of the dream, so you can experience awareness more often than you would otherwise.

Time Reminders

A meditative reminder is something you choose in the physical world to help you to return to awareness and presence. For the reminder to work, you need to empower a neural pathway that will remind you, and you need to follow through whenever it reminds you to be meditatively aware.

A great example of a reminder is a clock. When I was a middle school teacher in Japan, I had to look at the clock multiple times during a lesson for pacing purposes, so it became the perfect reminder for me.

Each time that I looked at the clock, I became spherically aware. As I had to look at the clock multiple times per lesson, and as I had on average four lessons per day, that added up to a lot of reminders and a lot of meditation time.

When I was in the Teachers' Room, I used the time indicator on my computer and the clock on the wall for reminders. Each time I saw a timepiece, I tried to take a moment to at least flash into calm spherical awareness. You should do the same.

For awareness reminders to work, it is important you first program your mind to remind you each time you check the time. The way to do that is as follows:

1. Look at the time. Flash into a relaxed spherical awareness and maintain it until you feel like you are in a meditated state.
2. As soon as you feel you are in a meditated state, look away from the timepiece and intentionally focus your mind to come back to a non-meditated state.
3. Look at the time again and flash back into spherical awareness.
4. Once meditated, look away and focus the mind to come back to a focused beta brain wave.
5. Repeat the process at least 5-10 times.

Once you believe you have successfully set your reminder, you need to test it to be sure it works. To test the reminder, forget about meditation and go about your usual daily activity. If the reminder works, the next time you check the time, you will remember to meditate. If the reminder failed, it means you need to spend a little more time programming the reminder into your mind.

Once a reminder is programmed, you must maintain the association to keep the reminder working. Even if you can meditate only briefly whenever you see the time, know that that time stimulates your brain to remap, to allow for greater ease with awareness henceforth. If you do not meditate when you see the time, then you are undoing the association.

Asymmetry Reminders

One of my students, Barbara, came up with a nifty reminder strategy that I would like to share with you. She cleverly began altering things around her house so that they would serve as reminders. For example, she would turn a vase upside down, so that whenever she entered the room, the vase would catch her eye, which would remind her to meditate. You could do the same thing with pictures, by intentionally tilting one of them so that it catches your eye. Each time you see it, you have been reminded to meditate.

You could slightly alter positioning and direction of furniture, so that the asymmetry pulls your attention. That's a great reminder. Each time you notice the asymmetry, you will meditate. If you have other people living in the house, who don't want you messing with things in this way, see if you can make the changes so subtle that you will notice but they will not. That very intention will get you to notice extremely subtle changes.

If you just can't stand a tiny asymmetry, note that the force within that feels disturbed is not in alignment with relaxed spherical awareness. See if you can soften the resistance through exposure, much like you learned to accept a cold shower. If you need a gradual approach to overcome the resistance to asymmetries in your house, you might make tiny asymmetries you will notice but that will not bother you so. As you gain acceptance of a little asymmetry, you could intentionally increase the asymmetry as a challenge. Mentor your mind and body with awareness.

Asymmetry Game

If you have a partner who is willing to aid in your meditative process, you could make game of it by having them slightly alter something different in the house each day, but without telling you what they altered until the end of the day.

As a part of the game, you know they altered something, and that knowledge will inspire you to keep an eye out for it. The curiosity alone will remind you to meditate more, and, of course, when you find the alteration, you will meditate as you correct the imbalance.

At the end of the day, check with your partner to see if you correctly noticed the one thing that they changed. The feedback they give you will help you to measure your progress with awareness.

If you fail to notice what they changed time and again, they will need to make the changes a little more obvious. If you notice easily what they change, then they should make the changes a little more subtle. You want to be right at the edge of your awareness abilities, so you are constantly being challenged.

If your partner is kindly moving things around in the house to remind you to meditate, then each time you find what they moved, be sure to meditate, even if only briefly, then move the reminding object back to its original position. If you don't correct the object's position, before long, your house will be utterly disorganized, which would be unhelpful.

Chapter 20

The Heart of Chaos

Most of us, when we think of chaos, reflect on the unpredictable, changing world around us. We understand that to survive, we humans must either adapt to our environment or try to control our environment so that it fits with us. Of course, all animals, by their very existence, affect their environment, but they do so without a plan.

That is not to say that animals have no capacity to plan. Some animals clearly demonstrate the ability to plan and strategize. Crows, ravens, and magpies, for example, can pick up a stick and fashion it to fish ants out of an ant hill. That sequence of actions seems to demonstrate an ability to plan a strategy and fashion a tool to execute that strategy. These birds seem to fashion tools consciously. We can see similar abilities in simians and the great apes. Likely, many animals have some degree of conscious strategizing.

Human beings, however, have taken the ability to plan and fashion our environment far beyond the rest of the animal kingdom. But even with our incredible abilities for planning and execution, most of us can't set a simple aim for self-improvement and follow through on it for more than a few weeks. How is it that we can almost completely transform our external environments, but are seemingly inept at improving our inner lives?

The answer is that there is an inner force within you that does not want to change, that does not want to improve, that does not want you to reach your true potential. That inner force is your greatest enemy, disguised as your greatest ally. We will call that force "The Deceiver."

The Deceiver is the true heart of chaos in your life. The Deceiver speaks seductively through unhealthy avoidances, urges, and compulsion, which we may experience with some regularity every day.

Where does that voice come from? Where is its throne? If you could find that throne, you would find The Deceiver sitting there. Once you find The Deceiver, could you usurp it and take your rightful place of authority in your life? If you could, then you could set a wise goal and follow through without hesitation or inner resistance. If that happened, the war within would end, and you would be at peace.

Have you noticed The Deceiver in your life? If not, do you want to notice it? If you don't want to see it yet, that is fine. With practice, at some point down the road, you will naturally be ready to notice, and at that time, you may want to revisit this chapter.

Discovering the Deceiver

If you would like to become aware of The Deceiver, here is how to take the first step toward a powerful transformation.

Most people who train themselves via the TEM cold shower method, eventually notice an odd phenomenon. You too are likely to notice it before too long. After a few weeks or months of daily practice, you will notice that while taking the shower, you enjoy it more than warm showers. The fact that cold showers become more enjoyable than warm showers is strange enough, but there is something stranger still you may start to notice. Here's what typically happens.

Even though you enjoy cold showers more than warm showers, during the lead up to taking your daily shower, you notice that there is still some sort of inner resistance to taking cold showers. It's a baffling experience because it's as if there are two yous. One of you seems to enjoy the cold showers and wants to move toward a better quality of life by taking on healthy challenges and responsibilities. That you is refreshing and inspiring. The other "you" seems to hate the cold showers for reasons that are not immediately obvious or rational.

From repeated experience, you know you enjoy the cold showers while experiencing them, so why would there be resistance prior to taking them? And why does that resistance seem to disappear as soon as the cold water hits your skin? Not only does it disappear, for many people, it is replaced by vibrant awareness and a certain pleasure.

What the hell is creating the resistance? That is the question!

This is one of the most important questions you can possibly ask yourself, for when you have explored that question and realized the answer within your own body, you have discovered the force within that has been holding you back. You have discovered the cause of your ignorance and suffering. You have discovered that which all true sages discover. And once you have transcended that force, you find harmony within.

Can you define the nature of The Deceiver? Do you know what it is?

Transforming the Deceiver

In ancient times, people sought to exorcise evil spirits. It may seem a tempting idea, and you may want to get rid of The Deceiver in a similar fashion. I suggest that that approach is not going to be so productive, however, because removing The Deceiver would be like cutting out half of your brain. Instead of removing it, it's better to transform it, to make this contentious part of the self your greatest ally in service to life improvement, which is ultimately what it is meant to be.

The next time you get into the shower, stand in front of the shower knob directly under the showerhead, looking at it with the intention of turning it to the coldest setting that it can produce, while feeling for any signs of The Deceiver. Notice any tension, hesitation, anxiety, or any other negative feelings. Notice if you feel any anxiety, no matter how small. The feelings could be as simple as a tension in the breath, taking some sort of stance, or even a preparatory breath. All of that may be coming from The Deceiver, who is creating the illusion that the cold shower is going to be unpleasant even though you know it is not.

Once you notice the signs of The Deceiver, see if you can find where it is centered in the body. Most people will notice that it is located at the center of the diaphragm, a muscle that controls your breathing. It curves around just below your breastbone and beneath the ribcage in the front of your body.

Still looking at the shower head, ready to turn on the cold, notice the feeling and pinpoint it by touching the spot with your fingertip. As soon as you do that, turn the water on, with the aim of softening and releasing anxiety, fear, and negativity. Stand there under the shower head until the anxiety is gone, which for most people will be almost instantly. Turn the shower off and stand there for 15 or 20 seconds.

Next look at the showerhead again with the determination of doing a second round. Notice if there is any hesitation or anxiety. If there is, put your finger on the spot where you feel it in the body. As soon as you touch it, turn on the shower again for another dousing. Release all resistance until you are smiling broadly. Repeat this process over and over until all hesitation is absolutely gone.

For safety's sake, if you notice shivering or any other signs of hypothermia as they are listed in Chapter 17, even if there is still some hesitation, call it a day, but with the determination that you will repeat the same process the next day.

The next day, when you take your cold shower, see if you can follow the One Breath guideline as is found in Chapter 14. The basic idea is that you take no preparatory steps other than meditating and removing your clothing. Within one breath of stepping into the shower, step directly under the shower head and turn it on without any tension whatsoever.

As you move forward each day, a little less tethered to the negative power of The Deceiver, your life begins to improve tremendously. Be sure not to develop a negative outlook on The Deceiver, for condemnation is an attitude of The Deceiver. If condemnation is motivating you, be aware you have been duped again. Don't feel bad about it, though, because that feeling does not help, a sign that it too is The Deceiver. It's a genius in its games, and you will not outsmart it. Of course, you are welcome to try—I know I have tried plenty of times.

Soften any negativity, return to spherical awareness, and move forward with a gentle smile. That is the way.

Chapter 21

Daily Embodiment

Many of us have so much clutter in our physical, emotional, and mental lives that we simply do not know where to begin making corrections. When we look at all the areas of our lives that are out of balance, we may feel overwhelmed, especially when we think about how long it might take to make those corrections. The big picture view may not be very encouraging. The great news is you don't have to correct your entire life. All you need to do is get this day right according to four basic guidelines–what is necessary, helpful, engaging, and meaningful.

As you have probably noticed, lack of awareness leaves you vulnerable to urges and compulsions. Awareness leads you toward that which is necessary, helpful, engaging, and meaningful according to your own definitions. The key to embodying awareness in daily life is not found in correcting your entire life today, but in simply getting this day right. If, today, you are heading more toward that which is in alignment with those four guidelines, then you are making progress. Of course, as you move forward, your definitions of those four criteria will begin to refine as awareness increases in your life. With experience, you will start to notice that some of the things you thought were engaging, meaningful, helpful, and necessary, are no longer meeting the criteria. The refinement of your criteria is a natural part of the awareness process. As your criteria refine, so too does your awareness increase.

To get your day right, you need to get the moment right, which will require a little bit of awareness. This chapter provides you with a basic template to help you to get more of your moments right, which will then help you to get your day heading in the right direction, according to your own definitions.

Wake up!

When you wake up in the morning, is your head clear, or are you in a prolonged mental fog? Do you immediately leap out of bed, or do you press snooze and roll over again hoping for a little more sleep? Most of us make liberal use of snooze and are in a somewhat dazed state for the better part of an hour upon waking. The tendency is understandable considering our lifestyles.

If you were a Samurai, would the prolonged foggy condition be acceptable to you? If you were a hunter-gatherer, would that condition be helpful to your survival and that of your tribe? I hope you answered "no" to those questions.

Instinctively, we know that the snooze button and the morning fog are not compatible with a life lived close to the earth. Reflecting on our dazed condition a little, we can easily see that it results from being insulated from the pressures of nature. Any wild animal that follows such a disconnected, unaware pattern is unlikely to survive long enough to reproduce.

Modern humans are the result of billions of years of evolution, the continuation of genetics that survived all the pressures of life long enough to successfully procreate. The fact that you are alive in this moment seems to be the result of the most amazing lottery ever played.

Scientist Dr. Ali Binazir ran a thought experiment that sheds a bit of fun light on the odds of your existence (Spector). Although there is no way to be sure of his numbers, the experiment should make you take your life a little less for granted.

Dr. Binazir begins by assuming that the chance of your parents meeting was one in 20,000 because 20,000 women are about what the average male is likely to encounter over 25 years of his life. The next assumption is that after your parents met, that they committed to each other long enough to have you, a chance that Dr. Binazir estimates at one in 2000. Combining these two sets of calculations brings our chances of existing to one in 40 million—a small chance indeed, but he takes it further.

Dr. Binazir then estimates that the average woman has about 100,000 eggs and the average man produces about four trillion sperm cells. He calculates that the one right sperm meeting the one right egg that would produce you faces odds of one in four quadrillion, or 4,000,000,000,000,000.

By that number, it seems your existence is a miracle of miracles, but still the number is too small, because this number only takes into account your parents meeting and reproducing. It overlooks the four billion years of evolutionary generations that proceeded you, going all the way back to the first single-celled organism, all of which had the tiniest odds of passing on the exact combination of genetic material required for you to ever be born.

You might disagree with these estimates. You might think that the chances of your parents meeting were half of what he estimated (10,000) and that the chances of them procreating was half as well (1000), but even by halving the numbers, your chances of existing would be roughly 1 in 100 million. And that is if we only take one generation into account.

To get the big picture, we need to toss in the four billion years of evolution where those same odds affected the chance of existence of every single generation leading up to your birth. The final number that Dr. Binazir came up with is 1 in 10 to the 2,685,000th power, a number that far exceeds all the estimated atoms of the entire universe, which is estimated at 10 to the 80th power.

How do the chances of your birth relate to waking up dazed in the morning? Your very existence is predicated upon all the generations leading up to our modern safe world not waking up groggy. Waking up sharp is a genetic priority for survival. When you wake up dull, inevitably you are going to feel much more anxiety, frustration, and weakness throughout your day because your nervous system is thrown off-kilter. It instinctively knows that being in a prolonged fog is genetic suicide.

The question is this: how do we wake up sharp as a tack, ready to take on the would-be assassin in the room or the task of getting children up and out the door on time in a harmonious way or handle that business meeting in the best way possible? The answer: we need a powerful motivation to get up immediately upon waking.

Take a squirrel, for example: if it had the option to sleep in every day and still have enough food, chances are it would hit snooze too if it could. Nature provides the motivation for the other animals' wakefulness. If you lived in a debris hut in the middle of the forest, you would wake up sharp, as a squirrel does.

Because you don't have the natural forces to wake you up, you need to provide the motivation yourself. Think about a time in your life when you sprang out of bed sharp as a tack. Chances are that in the moment you woke up, your mind recalled something important that needed to be done instantly. Fortunately, to wake up sharp and on time you can use instinct.

Here is a game you can play that will help you to wake up in Samurai fashion. Before you go to sleep, set an intention to imagine the following scenario as soon as you wake up: there is a stranger in the room, and you need to get up immediately to protect yourself and your family.

The more vivid you can make the intention the night before, the more vividly will it spring to mind when you wake up. The first few nights you try this, when you wake up, you may not remember the scenario, but after several nights of setting the intention, it will happen.

If you don't like imagining a home intruder, you can try other methods. The basic idea is to create some sort of life structure that gets you out of bed in the morning—a detailed plan of action for the first hour of your day. I personally find teaching online TEM guided meditations each morning to be a powerful motivation for a quick wakeup. As an author who sets my own schedule, without such a commitment I could easily get up whenever I wanted to, which would negatively affect my health and awareness, as well as ruin the overall quality of my day.

Absent the survival demands of nature, we need to have a powerful purpose to get up. If you don't have one naturally, you need to construct one. Once you get into the pattern of waking up early and sharp, a pattern that can take several weeks to engrain, your body will feel comparatively better throughout the day. You will be healthier and likely sleep better at night, which will further help you wake up clear-minded and ready for activity.

If all else fails, at least move your alarm clock out of arm's reach, so you must get out of bed to turn it off. If the snooze option is easy, it might prove too tempting to your untrained morning self.

The Bathroom

Once up out of bed, do not allow yourself to get back in. Instead, head directly to the bathroom to release your bladder and meditatively visit with your teacher, the cold.

Once you are done urinating, open a window to allow in the fresh air. From a meditated state, feel and smell the crispness of the air. Observe the world around you.

If you are going to practice primary sounds, you might want to close the window so you do not disturb your neighbors, if you have any.

Take your cold shower or bath in a meditated state. Smile.

Exiting the Bathroom

Leave the bathroom in a state of spherical awareness. Feel your house and use your X-Ray Vision.

Move silently in awareness as if you were checking for an intruder. See if you can notice where family members are and what they are doing before you physically see them. Make it fun.

If you are a coffee or tea drinker, try not standing and staring dully as the beverage brews, an incredible waste of time. Instead, pay attention to the entire space around you while doing something productive.

Consider weaning yourself off the caffeine habit, so you are no longer reliant on a substance to wake up. I love coffee, too.

The Day

Go about your day being attentive to the reminders you set. Each time you spontaneously remember to meditate or notice a reminder, be sure to become spherically aware even if only for a minute.

Whenever you enter spherical awareness, see if you can reduce the amount of effort the transition requires and see if you can maintain that state for a bit longer.

As you go about your day, notice The Deceiver, who justifies, delays, avoids, criticizes, and condemns. Each time you notice that energy, soften the inner space and return to spherical awareness.

Going to sleep

Before getting into bed, take an accounting of your day. What sort of urges and compulsions did you experience? Did you go along with them or not? What, if anything, did you do that was engaging but not meaningful? Did you participate in any unhelpful habits and distractive comforts? Such activities are not born of awareness.

Before you go to sleep, make a plan to do more of that which is engaging and meaningful, helpful, and necessary by your own definitions, not compulsive comforts. Comfort has its season. Within proper measure, comfort is necessary and meaningful, but comfort should not be running your life.

Did you accomplish all the things you aimed to do? Ask this question without shame, guilt, or blame, for those energies are not born of awareness, so they will not serve your benevolent aims for a better life.

After reflecting on your day, set your aim to wake up sharp and spend a little bit more time in awareness than you did today. Finally, keep your training light and fun. Make this process an adventure. Don't get too serious.

Chapter 22

Transformation

A strange thing happens when we test the stability of our meditative practices under pressure like we do with TEM training. Initially the challenges may seem impossible, but with persistence, we soon discover that the quality of our lives begins to improve. We see that we have more energy, are more inspired, and we get more done. Simply put, we feel better, and that positive feeling seems to spiral out into the world around us.

With repeated practice over the span of a few months, most practitioners will find that they can easily produce all primary sounds without any noticeable wavering–A, I, U, E, O, M, and N. By this time, most people are enjoying cold showers so much that they wash their bodies in cold showers, only using hot water to wash their hair.

Usually within a month of cold showers, individuals are ready to begin testing visual awareness meditation within the shower, and, shortly thereafter, spherical awareness. Eventually, they notice The Deceiver and begin working to soften and release the fear that fuels that inner force.

With persistence, it won't take long before you are able to meditate with relative ease anywhere you are; you will see you can even meditate while walking, while running or doing any number of other strenuous activities. Awareness becomes an integral part of your daily life. Most importantly, you can wake up and go to sleep with a smile on your face because you just feel good.

In the process of the training, you are likely to notice you stop putting off doing things that need to be done, because you see that each time you avoid doing what is necessary, you accumulate a kind of psychic debt, and that debt weighs on you. Noticing the price you pay for delaying responsibility, you start taking care of things immediately, and that frees your mind.

As the mind is freed of psychic debt, you have access to more energy and inspiration, which naturally leads you to face fears, traumas, and other inner blockages that have been holding you back. As those fears and inner blockages soften, you naturally feel attracted to the idea of taking on greater and greater responsibility for no other reason than it feels good to do so.

With practice, you will also notice you no longer fall prey as often to urges and compulsions. You notice also that you feel more inclined to be honest with yourself and with others. You are no longer inclined to submit to people in an attempt to be liked or to dominate them in an attempt to feel power. As our energy strengthens, inner clarity emerges, while anxiety wanes.

With persistent, sincere, but playful practice, you will begin to notice that other people treat you differently. New opportunities may begin to open to you because other people will see you have a certain admirable quality. Some people may tell you that they would like to be a little more like you, and some of them will even ask you for advice on how to improve their lives.

A natural confidence emerges that has nothing to do with identity or how people think of you. This confidence is the bane of toxic personalities. Quite naturally, some people will try to prevent your continued progress, so you will be the person that they perhaps used to be able to control. Still others will begin to move away from you. You might let them go without any ill feelings toward them, or maybe you will hold on by pretending you are still the person that they can control. It's your life; it's up to you. That said, once you have enough awareness to clearly see the nature of The Deceiver, you'll probably move toward greater health regardless of what others want from you or think about you, which means you will be free of their control mechanisms.

With persistence, you might start to feel like a whole new person, transformed through daily TEM training. At that time, you will understand why the old "you" felt so ineffectual and weak, but you will no longer feel like that person. Furthermore, you will be able to look at other people and see within them the same thing that was holding you back—The Deceiver.

Even if after sincere, long-term training, The Deceiver is still there, you will see that it is softening and resisting your wise aims noticeably less than it did before you began TEM training. Because you experience less inner resistance, less inner chaos, life feels so much easier to deal with. The improvement you see will keep you moving forward in awareness regardless of external life circumstances. At some point, you will realize you simply can't go back to life as you lived it before TEM training, because that way of life is no longer interesting to you.

If you keep up the training, within a year or two, your whole life will likely be transformed for the better, not just because external circumstances changed for the better, but because from the abundance of your heart something beautiful and healthy flows into the world. All of this came about because you decided to challenge your meditative awareness with cold showers and daily life practice.

Remember, if you apply the tools found in this book to transcend the resistances you experience in daily life, nothing can hold you back, for you have already gone a long way toward overcoming your greatest challenge, the war within. There is no greater challenge in this world than that.

Keep up your training!

Your friend in awareness,
Richard L. Haight
June 10, 2020

Ready Reference

Balancing the Brain Hemispheres through Neuroplasticity (Chapter 1)

Whatever you can do with your dominant hand, practice doing with your non-dominant hand, aiming to equalize your abilities between left and right hands. Great exercises include writing, drawing, eating, brushing teeth, brushing hair, carrying things, throwing, batting, bowling, et cetera.

Vagal Breathing (Chapter 2)

1. Sit down to keep you safe in case you faint.
2. Take in a full breath and hold it while tensing your entire body. Be sure to tense the face slightly as well. Hold the tension along with the breath.
3. Although it may seem as if your lungs are full, that is not actually the case. Without exhaling the current air in your lungs, inhale again to fully top off your lungs.
4. Hold the air and physical tension for as long as you can.
5. When you can no longer hold your breath, exhale slowly and relax the body. Allow your body to breathe naturally.

Feeling Primary Sounds (Chapter 5)

1. Sit up or stand straight but comfortably.
2. Relax the body and defocus the mind while feeling the entire physical body.
3. Begin vocalizing "Ah" while feeling the vibrations in the body for a few seconds. Note the shape and direction of vibrational travel.
4. Shift the sound to "Ee" for a few seconds and note the vibrational change in shape as compared to making the "Ah" sound. Notice the direction that the sound travels.
5. Continuing, change the sound to "Ew" for a brief duration. Feel and note the shape and direction of sound travel as compared to the "Ee" sound.
6. Shift into the "Eh" sound and note the change, the shape, and the travel of the sound.
7. Change to the "Oh" sound and feel its qualities.
8. Make the "Mmm" sound and note its nature.
9. Finally, produce the "Nnn" sound and feel its dimensions.
10. Produce them all in one breath, while feeling the change between them–"Ah," "Ee," "Ew," "Eh," "Oh," "Mmm," and "Nnn."

Sound Sensitivity (Chapter 6)

Make all the sounds "Ah," "Ee," "Ew," "Eh," "Oh," "Mmm" and "Nnn" while feeling the entire body. Note which sounds feel the most pleasant and the least pleasant to the body.

Sound Therapy (Chapter 6)

1. Try each sound while feeling the body's response–"Ah," "Ee," "Ew," "Eh," "Oh," "Mmm" and "Nnn."

2. The sound that is therapeutic, at this time, will feel somehow right or fulfilling to your body.
3. Practice the sound that produces the most positive feeling for 5 to 10 minutes.

Breath of Fire (Chapter 8)

- Used at the start of a cold shower to get your breathing under control.
- Intentionally guide convulsive breathing into rapid, full, powerful inhales and exhales.

Testing the Power of Cold Showers (Chapter 8)

1. Wait until you feel negative or otherwise emotional.
2. Head into your bathroom, strip off your clothes, and step into a stream of the coldest water your shower can provide with the intention that the shocking embrace of the cold water washes away the negativity.
3. Stand completely under the flowing water for at least a minute using Breath of Fire.
4. Direct the water to your face, over your head, chest, back–to the places that cause your breathing to constrict the most.
5. Try not to escape the stream in any way.
6. After you get your breathing under control, aim to relax.
7. Intentionally release negativity with your breath.
8. After one minute, turn off the water, step out of the shower, and dry your body.
9. Notice how you feel.

First Training Shower (Chapter 8)

1. Set a timer for 10 minutes to remind you to get out prior to cold shower training.
2. To get the maximum benefit of a cold shower, do it first thing in the morning after using the toilet.
3. With as little thought as possible, strip off your clothes, step into the shower, and if you can get yourself to do it, position yourself fully under the faucet.
4. Turn the water on to the strongest, coldest setting possible.
5. Notice any flinch responses or unstable breathing.
6. During the first minute use Breath of Fire to gain control of your breathing, while directing the flow of the water directly to the places that stimulate the most breathing tension.
7. Once past the first minute, aim to stay in the cold shower for as long as you can, but no more than 10 minutes.

Gradual Approach (Chapter 8)

1. Direct the shower stream first to your feet, then gradually up your legs, to your crotch, then to your lower abdomen. You might also direct the spray up your arms before finally aiming the stream at your torso, face, head, shoulders, and down your back.
2. Mentally note the time you were in the cold stream, and, if you were able to regulate your breathing, roughly how long it took to smooth it out.
3. Once your shower is complete, immediately dry yourself.

The Sink Method (Chapter 8)

1. Put your head under the sink faucet and run cold water over your head.

2. Use your hand to direct the faucet water over your face and neck.
3. Keep up this process for at least a minute.
4. When done with the head, face, and neck, run the cold water over your arms.
5. Once you are done with the water, hold your head above the sink for a few minutes to let the water drip off and be exposed to the air in the room.
6. Notice your breathing. You might note that you have breath releases every now and again, in which your body naturally sucks in a large breath and releases it in an invigorating way.
7. Dry yourself and go about your day.

Raynaud's Syndrome and Cold Showers (Chapter 9)

1. Take cold showers while standing in hot or warm bath water.
2. As soon as the shower is complete, sink into the warm bath to rapidly heat up your core temperature, which will get blood back into the ill-affected areas.

For extreme cases:

1. First fill up the bath with hot water and bathe until your body is filled with heat.
2. Once the body battery is charged with heat, stand up in the warm water and turn on the cold shower. Doing this, you will find that the cold is not nearly so shocking because your body is radiating such heat.
3. Once you are finished with the shower, if you have any signs of Raynaud's activation, lie back down in the bath to warm up.

Other Disabilities (Chapter 9)

1. Using your sink or a bucket of cold water, wet a washcloth and use it to spread the cold water over every area of your body that you can.
2. Continually re-wet it with cold water as you go about wiping your body to maintain the cold temperature.
3. Once you have wet your body, air dry yourself. Any resulting Raynaud's symptoms are a good indicator you need to skip the air-drying.
4. During the air dry, you will likely notice shivering and nipple constriction. That is fine.
5. If you have any other symptoms of hypothermia, be sure to immediately towel off and put your clothes back on.

Measuring Progress through Primary Sounds (Chapter 10)

1. Just before entering the shower take a full breath and begin loudly vocalizing the primary sounds of "Ah" to get a baseline for the stability of the sound when not under pressure.
2. Be sure to open your mouth enough that the sound resonates sufficiently, but don't blast it out so loud that it annoys family members.
3. Continue chanting the sound until your lungs are empty.
4. Once you have your baseline for your primary sound, enter the shower, take another breath, and begin producing your sound.
5. Immediately turn on the water and aim it to run over your head, chest, and back, especially the areas that are most challenging.
6. Notice any wavering of the primary sound.
7. Each day aim to make the same full bodied, lengthy sounds in the cold shower as you did prior to taking the cold shower.
8. Notice that any lung contractions can be easily heard and felt when chanting.

9. When you find you can make a perfect "Ah," sound, the next challenge would be to try the "Oh" sound.
10. Once you can produce a solid "Oh" sound, move onto the "Mmm" sound and see how that goes.
11. With mastery of the "Mmm" sound, try the "Eh" sound, the "Ew" and "Ee" sounds to find which is the next proper challenge. Don't forget the "Nnn" sound.

Learning the Relationship between Energy Levels and Resistance (Chapter 11)

1. Take your cold shower at a time of day when you are at or near peak energy.
2. Notice the degree of mental and physical resistance you feel immediately prior to turning on the water when you are at peak energy.
3. Notice the degree of discomfort you feel in the shower and the length of time you can remain in the cold water as compared to when you shower first thing in the morning.

Experiment: Charging the Body with Heat (Chapter 11)

1. First thing in the morning, get up, head into the bathroom, and fill up the bathtub with hot water to your liking.
2. Take care of your toilet necessities, and then when the bath is full, take off your clothes, and get in.
3. Remain in the warm water for five or ten minutes to fully warm up your core body temperature.
4. Once your body is charged with warmth, drain the water, stand up, and get under the shower head.
5. Turn it on to full cold and see how your body reacts to the cold as compared with times when you did not charge the body with heat.

Transcending Resistant Mental Dialogues (Chapter 11)

1. Notice when resistance arises and the mental narrative that accompanies it.
2. Notice how one inner force aims to do what is healthy and another inner force seems aimed at avoiding discomfort.
3. Notice which forces predict our actions and inactions, for those forces represent our deepest patterns, many of which may need to be softened if we are to make real progress.
4. Support the healthy inner forces by consistently following through with their aims.

Mentoring Your Way through Resistive Mental Dialogues (Chapter 12)

1. When you notice any internal narrative that is resistant to the cold shower, see if it feels like it is your voice. If it feels like your voice, it means you are identified with your thoughts and emotions, which means you think they are you.
2. Pause, relax, and totally defocus your mind.
3. Once relaxed and defocused, try using the sink method you learned in Chapter 8.
4. You may find you are able to use that method because it represents a pleasant step down from the threat of the cold shower, which the resistive inner force was so focused on avoiding.
5. Once your vagal nerve is stimulated from the sink method, consider the shower again. Would you be willing to get your feet wet? Chances are that the answer is "Yes."
6. Get in the shower and get your feet wet without any thought beyond that step.
7. Hold the cold water on your feet for a bit, and then ask yourself if you could try aiming the water at your lower legs. You'll likely discover that you can.

8. Now try your upper legs.
9. Keep going until you finally reach a place where you are simply not willing to go any further. If you hit what feels like an impenetrable blockage, stop, get out, and call it a day.
10. The next day, do the same process and see how far you can get. Chances are that within a week or two, you will be able to take the full shower without nearly as much inner resistance.
11. The next step in dealing with the unhelpful inner force is to see if you can now directly enter the shower and speed up the process of the cold water exposure by making it a flowing progression instead of a step-by-step process.
12. With persistence over a period of days or weeks, it will only take you 10-20 seconds to get the water up to your head.
13. Once you get to that point, the next step is to see how long you can remain in the cold shower.
14. Stop before the resistance gets too strong.
15. Eventually, wean yourself of gradual approaches.

Starting out Lukewarm (Chapter 13)

1. Get into the shower with the intention of first using lukewarm water and slowly turning it toward cold as you acclimate physically and mentally during the session.
2. Over a period of days, you will be able to apply gradually colder showers.

Mentoring Your Way through Skittishness (Chapter 13)

1. Notice when your body does not seem to want to face the shower.
2. Notice feelings of avoidance such as wanting to go back to sleep or maybe desiring to change your morning routine to postpone the shower.

3. Experience the feeling for a moment to get to know its presence, then defocus your mind and meditate yourself to calm awareness.
4. Once calm and centered in awareness, get in touch with the energy or force within you that truly wants you to become stronger, healthier, and more aware.
5. Once in touch with the benevolent force, ask yourself whether taking a cold shower is better for you than not taking one.
6. If you are tapped into benevolence, that which aims to fulfill your full potential as a human being, you will know when you are subconsciously trying to escape discomfort or when there is a valid reason to skip or postpone the shower on that day.

Applying the One Breath Principle (Chapter 14)

Whenever you have a good idea or plan of action, within the span of one breath, take some form of physical action to help birth the thought or plan into the world such as writing your ideas in a pocket notebook.

Visual Awareness Meditation (Chapter 15)

1. Set a timer to 15 minutes.
2. Sit comfortably with your eyes open, without bulging them.
3. Defocus your mind and gaze straight ahead with the aim of viewing the entire visual field.
4. To be sure you are seeing the entire visual field, without moving your eyes, make a mental note of a place or object on the right side that marks the very edge of your visual field.
5. Find markers for the left side, as well as the highest and lowest points that you can see.
6. Remain visually aware of the entire visual field.
7. Relax the entire body, but especially the eyes, lips, jaw, neck, shoulders, hands, and your breathing.

8. Note differences between foveal (focused) and peripheral (defocused) vision in terms of how each practice makes your body feel. What are the advantages of each visual mode, as you experience it?
9. After 15 minutes of seated visual awareness meditation, challenge your meditation by looking around with defocused eyes.
10. Try moving an arm or a leg.
11. Try getting up and sitting down again.
12. Try walking around.

Meditating Under Pressure (Chapter 15)

1. Set a timer for 10 minutes to remind you to get out prior to cold shower training.
2. Prior to entering the bathroom, get yourself into a meditated state via the visual awareness meditation.
3. Relax the body and mind deeply without thinking about the shower.
4. If you can, get in the shower without a single thought of the cold water.
5. Be sure you are still meditated before starting the shower.
6. See if you can turn on the water while maintaining physical and mental relaxation.
7. Keep the eyes unfocused.
8. If you find your mind or body tenses with anticipation when you look at the shower knob, then you know it is the fear and anticipation of discomfort that has pulled you out of primary awareness.
9. Notice what the mind does. There is nothing special you need to do about the tension other than to relax the body and defocus the mind again while gazing at the shower knob.

10. Once relaxed, begin your shower by directing the cold water flow to your feet via the gradual approach you learned in Chapter 8.
11. Whenever you feel your meditation break or weaken, redirect the shower head away and get back into the meditation before returning to the gradual process.
12. Go as far as you can while remaining meditated.
13. Try to remain in a meditated state while aiming the shower head at your face and closing your eyes. Remember to relax as much as possible and remain mentally defocused.
14. Be sure you are in conscious alpha (meditative awareness) when you exit the shower.
15. Dry yourself and get dressed while in meditation.
16. Exit the bathroom and see how long you can go through your daily activities while aware.

Spherical Awareness Meditation (Chapter 16)

1. While looking straight ahead, briefly flash your attention to your left side without physically looking there.
2. Now do the same thing with your right side.
3. Try it again while being attentive behind you.
4. Do it one more time in each direction rapidly, left, right, behind, up, and down.
5. Now try it again, but with relaxation.
6. See how long you can remain in a relaxed spherical awareness.

Pressure-Training Spherical Awareness (Chapter 16)

1. Set a timer for 10 minutes to remind you to get out prior to cold shower training.
2. Be sure you are in spherical awareness prior to entering the cold bath.

3. See if you can step in and sit down in one seamless, aware, harmonious motion that flows from one motion to the next without pause or haste.
4. Once seated, without pause or hurry, extend your legs to immerse them fully in the water.
5. Once your legs are fully wet, hold your breath and lie back as gracefully as possible to submerge your torso and head.
6. Remain submerged for as long as you can comfortably hold your breath, while in spherical awareness.
7. Once you are ready to take your next breath, sit up and fully relax in a deep meditation.
8. As you sit there, your body heat will warm the water near it, and that will create an insulative barrier from the coldest water. Every now and again use your hands and legs to gracefully move the water around so your body experiences the coldest temperatures available.
9. After a minute or so of sitting in meditation, with grace, hold your breath and re-submerge your upper body and head until you are ready to exhale.
10. At the ten-minute mark (or before if you are experiencing any symptoms of hypothermia), exit the bathtub gracefully in spherical awareness.
11. Dry off and get dressed, and continue your day in spherical awareness.

Once you get the hang of remaining spherically aware through the basic bath that I outlined above, forget the form, and do whatever feels right while you are in the cold bath. Feel your way through the experience from a deep spherical awareness.

Sick Days (Chapter 17)

1. If you are not feeling well one morning, you might omit the cold bath and even the cold shower and instead use only the sink method.
2. If your energy is extremely low, you have a fever, chills, or signs of sickness, avoid all forms of cold training as they can weaken your body even further. Take a rest on days like that.
3. If you are not feeling sick, but feel a bit low on energy, you might continue your training via the sink method detailed in Chapter 8.

Symptoms of Hypothermia (Chapter 17)

- Shivering
- Slurred speech or mumbling
- Slow, shallow breathing
- Weak pulse
- Clumsiness or lack of coordination
- Drowsiness or extremely low energy
- Confusion or memory loss
- Loss of consciousness

Hypothermia Risk Factors (Chapter 17)

- Fatigue or exhaustion will reduce your tolerance for cold.
- Older age can reduce the body's ability to regulate body temperature and to sense the symptoms of hypothermia.
- In adolescence the body loses heat faster than is common with adults.
- Mental problems such as dementia and other conditions may interfere with judgment or awareness of the symptoms of hypothermia as they set in.

- Alcohol causes the blood vessels to expand, which can make the body feel warm. Due to this expansion of the blood vessels when they should be contracting to protect from the cold, the body will lose heat more rapidly. Furthermore, alcohol diminishes the natural shivering response, which is one of the first signs that you need to get out of the water. With alcohol, there is also a risk of passing out in the water.
- Recreational drugs affect judgment and can lead to passing out in the cold water.
- Medical conditions that affect regulation of body temperature such as hypothyroidism, anorexia nervosa, diabetes, stroke, severe arthritis, Parkinson's disease, trauma, and spinal cord injuries increase the risk of hypothermia.
- Medications such as antidepressants, antipsychotics, pain medications, and sedatives can reduce the body's ability to regulate heat.

Cold Bath Meditation (Chapter 17)

1. Set a timer for 10 minutes to remind you to get out prior to cold shower training.
2. Be sure you are in spherical awareness prior to entering the cold bath.
3. See if you can step in and sit down in one seamless, aware, harmonious motion that flows from one movement to the next without pause or haste.
4. Once seated, without pause or haste, extend your legs to immerse them fully in the water.
5. Once your legs are fully wet, hold your breath and lie back as gracefully as possible to submerge your torso and head.
6. Remain submerged for as long as you can comfortably hold your breath, while in spherical awareness.

7. Once you are ready to take your next breath, sit up and fully relax in a deep meditation.
8. As you sit there, your body heat will warm the water near it, and that will create an insulative barrier from the coldest water. Every now and again use your hands and legs to gracefully move the water around so your body experiences the coldest temperatures available.
9. After a minute or so of sitting in meditation, with grace, hold your breath and re-submerge your upper body and head until you are ready to exhale.
10. At the ten-minute mark (or before if you are experiencing any symptoms of hypothermia), exit the bathtub gracefully in spherical awareness.
11. Dry off, get dressed, and continue your day in spherical awareness.
12. Once you get the hang of remaining spherically aware through the basic bath that I outlined above, forget the form, and do whatever feels right while you are in the cold bath. Feel your way through the experience from a deep spherical awareness.

X-Ray Vision (Chapter 18)

1. With open eyes, imagine you have X-Ray Vision that allows you to see through walls to the rooms, doors, hallways, et cetera that lay beyond your physical sight.
2. If you are outdoors, you could visualize the lay of the land, the trees, hills, rivers, et cetera, that are beyond your physical sight.
3. Create a low detail 3-D mental map of your surroundings such that if you closed your eyes, you could imagine the entire space that includes the obvious objects like furniture.

Spinning with X-Ray Vision (Chapter 18)

1. Stand up and look around you to create a mental map of your surroundings.
2. Once you have your surroundings mapped, extend your awareness over the entire area spherically as you have already learned to do.
3. Once awareness is extended, close your eyes while activating your imaginary X-Ray Vision, and begin to turn slowly in place like the hand of a clock.
4. While slowly turning with eyes closed, select an object like a room or a door to point out after you have taken several 360-degree rotations.
5. As soon as that room or object is lined up with your nose, stop and point to it with your eyes still closed.
6. Open your eyes to check your accuracy.

Topographical View (Chapter 18)

1. From a meditated state, imagine your "spiritual eye" rises from your body, high into the air, to look down upon the topography surrounding you.
2. As you move around, keep updating the topographical view.

Assassin Game (Chapter 18)

In this game, you will imagine that other people are assassins out to get you.

1. Expand your spherical awareness through the entire space of your home, for example, with the aim of sensing where other people are at all times.
2. To score a point, you need to notice someone approaching you before they come within 10 feet of you.

3. If someone approaches within 10 feet of you before you notice them, then you have been assassinated. In that case, your "opponent" scores a point.
4. At the end of each day, tally up how many times you avoided the assassination as compared to how many times you were assassinated.
5. Increase the challenge as you gain ability by adding more feet to the assassination distance.

Blind Spots (Chapter 18)

1. From a meditated state, start noticing where you look as you walk around your home, drive to and from work, and visit other frequented locations.
2. Notice the areas and things you look at consistently each time you move through the area. Also notice the places you tend to miss.
3. Once you start to perceive your own blind spots, take note of the blind spots of your family members and your neighbors.
4. Notice their regular patterns as well. For example, you might pay attention to the time that they tend to get the mail, take out the garbage, leave for work, return, et cetera.
5. Have fun!

Gateway Awareness (Chapter 18)

The purpose of this game is to remind you to be spherically aware and in the best possible position every time you move through a doorway or other narrow passage.

1. Use all doorways, hallways, or other such narrow spaces, including the ones at home, as triggers to reconnect with spherical awareness.
2. Try to be the last to enter or exit through any door or gateway.

Seat Positioning (Chapter 18)

1. Use spherical awareness to note the general layout of the building and the exits.
2. Notice which table provides the safest place to sit and observe.
3. Try to choose a table that has the fewest vectors of attack while simultaneously providing for best view of the entire space. A table in a corner provides the best possible vantage point without exposing your back.
4. Avoid sitting next to windows, doors, passageways, or the middle of the room.
5. If the ideal table is unavailable, aim for the next best table that provides a good view and relatively few vectors of attack.
6. Once you have found the best possible table, see if you can guide your group to sit there.
7. After moving to the selected table, you will want to sit in the most advantageous seat for your imaginary duties as a protector. That seat will allow optimal visual awareness of the entire space, while also allowing the best options for movement.

Alternative Exits (Chapter 18)

1. When in restaurants or other buildings, in spherical awareness, mentally map the layout of the place.
2. Make note of any openable windows and doors.
3. Glance into the kitchen to note if there is a back door.
4. Check the bathroom for a possible window you could use as an exit.

Time Reminders (Chapter 19)

1. Look at the time. Flash into a relaxed spherical awareness and maintain it until you feel like you are in a meditated state.
2. As soon as you feel you are in a meditated state, look away from the timepiece and intentionally focus your mind to come back to a non-meditated state.
3. Look at the time again and flash back into spherical awareness.
4. Once meditated, look away and focus the mind to come back to a focused beta brain wave.
5. Repeat the process at least 5-10 times.

Testing the Reminder (Chapter 19)

1. Once you have programmed your reminder, forget about meditation, and go about your usual daily activity.
2. If the reminder works, the next time you check the time, you will remember to meditate.
3. If the reminder failed, it means you need to spend a little more time programming the reminder into your mind.
4. Once a reminder is programmed, you must maintain the association to keep the reminder working.
5. The way to maintain the reminder is by meditating even if only briefly whenever you see the time.
6. If you do not meditate when you see the time, then you are undoing the association.

Asymmetry Reminders (Chapter 19)

1. Turn a vase upside down.
2. Intentionally tilt a wall photo or painting.
3. Slightly misalign furniture.

4. Each time you see the asymmetry, you have been reminded to meditate.

Asymmetry Game (Chapter 19)

1. Enlist family members and roommates to create asymmetries for you to find.
2. Correct asymmetries as you find them.
3. Check with the person at the end of each day to see whether you found their created asymmetry.
4. If the asymmetries are too subtle for you to notice, ask them to make them a bit more obvious.
5. If the asymmetries are easily noticed, you might ask them to make smaller adjustments as a challenge.

Transforming the Deceiver (Chapter 20)

1. Get into the shower, stand in front of the shower knob directly under the showerhead, while looking at it with the intention of turning it to the coldest setting that it can produce. Feel for any signs of The Deceiver.
2. Notice any tension, hesitation, anxiety, or any other negative feelings.
3. Notice if you feel any anxiety, no matter how small.
4. Once you notice the signs of The Deceiver, see if you can find where it is centered in the body.
5. Still looking at the shower head, ready to turn on the cold, notice the feeling, and pinpoint it by touching the spot with your fingertip.
6. Turn the water on, with the aim of softening and releasing anxiety, fear, and negativity.
7. Stand there under the shower head until the anxiety dissipates.
8. Turn the shower off and stand there for 15 or 20 seconds.

9. Look at the showerhead again with the determination of doing a second round.
10. Notice if there is any hesitation or anxiety.
11. Put your finger on the spot where you feel it in the body.
12. Turn on the shower again for another dousing.
13. Release all resistance until you are smiling broadly.
14. Repeat this process over and over until all hesitation is absolutely gone.

Note: if you notice shivering or any other signs of hypothermia as they are listed in Chapter 17, even if there is still some hesitation, call it a day, but with the determination that you will repeat the same process the next day.

Wake Up! (Chapter 21)

Ways to help you get up sharp and early:

- Before you go to sleep, set an intention to imagine that there is a stranger in the room, and you need to get up immediately to protect yourself and your family.
- Before you go to sleep, make a detailed plan of action for the first hour of your day.
- Move your alarm clock out of arm's reach, so you must get out of bed to turn it off.

The Bathroom (Chapter 21)

1. Once up out of bed, go directly to the bathroom to release your bladder and meditatively visit with your teacher, the cold.
2. Once you are done urinating, open a window to allow in the fresh air. From a meditated state, feel and smell the crispness of the air.
3. Observe the world around you.

4. If you are going to practice primary sounds, you might want to close the window so you do not disturb your neighbors, if you have any.
5. Take your cold shower or bath in a meditated state. Remember to smile!

Exiting the Bathroom (Chapter 21)

1. Exit the bathroom in a state of spherical awareness.
2. Feel your house and use your X-Ray Vision.
3. Move silently in awareness as if you were checking for an intruder.
4. See if you can notice where family members are and what they are doing before you physically see them. Make it fun.
5. If you are a coffee or tea drinker, while the beverage brews, pay attention to the entire space around you as you do something productive.

The Day (Chapter 21)

1. Go about your day being attentive to the reminders you set.
2. Each time you notice a trigger, be sure to become spherically aware even if only for a minute.
3. Whenever you enter spherical awareness, see if you can reduce the amount of effort it takes to do so and see whether you can maintain it for a bit longer.
4. As you go about your day, notice The Deceiver, who justifies, delays, avoids, criticizes, and condemns.
5. Each time you notice that energy, soften the inner space and return to spherical awareness.

Going to Sleep (Chapter 21)

1. Before getting into bed, take an accounting of your day.
   - What sort of urges and compulsions did you experience?
   - Did you go along with them or not?
   - What if anything did you do that was engaging but not meaningful?
   - Did you participate in any unhelpful habits and distractive comforts?
2. Before you go to sleep, make a plan to do more of that which is engaging, meaningful, helpful, and necessary by your own definitions, not compulsive comforts.
3. Set your aim to wake up sharp and spend a bit more time in awareness than you did today.
4. Be careful not to blame, shame, or guilt yourself. Keep the game light and fun.

The Warrior's Meditation Preview

The companion book to *Unshakable Awareness*

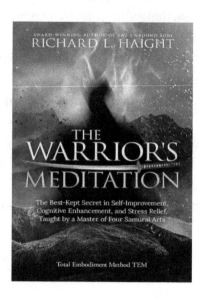

The Warrior's Meditation, by award-winning author of *The Unbound Soul,* Richard L. Haight, teaches the original, instinctive, non-religious form of meditation that has been all but lost to the world. Richard L. Haight, master of four Samurai arts, shares the best-kept secret in self-improvement, cognitive development, and stress-relief in the world.

For people of all backgrounds, genders, and ages

You may wonder how the Samurai's experience bears any resemblance to your modern life. After all, no armies or assassins seem to be trying to attack you or your town. In one way, we are not so different from the Samurai. With our busy lives, we don't have time to spend hours a day in meditation. Instead, we need a meditation that allows our actions in a high-pressure, fast-paced world to flow from a depth of awareness.

The Warrior's Meditation helps you access and express from that depth naturally.

The Warrior's Meditation is unlike any other meditation. This method is flexible in application, which allows it to blend with whatever your day has in store. Through short, daily sessions, the many scientifically verified cognitive and physical health benefits of daily meditation will open up to you through your active life. No longer do you need to retreat from life to meditate, for with *The Warrior's Meditation*, you can bring calm, clear awareness and vibrant life with you wherever you are. Eventually, you will fully embody meditation as a way of being, not just a doing.

Other Books by Richard L. Haight

The Unbound Soul: A Visionary Guide to Spiritual Transformation and Enlightenment

Inspirience: Meditation Unbound: The Unconditioned Path to Spiritual Awakening

The Psychedelic Path: An Exploration of Shamanic Plants for Spiritual Awakening

About the Author

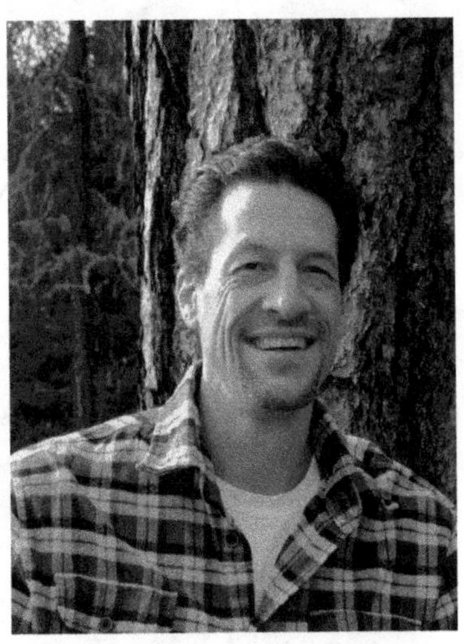

Richard L. Haight is the author of the bestselling titles *The Warrior's Meditation* and *The Unbound Soul*, and he is a master-level instructor of martial, meditation and healing arts. Richard began formal martial arts training at age 12 and moved to Japan the age of 24 to advance his training with masters of the sword, staff, and aiki-jujutsu.

During his 15 years living in Japan, Richard was awarded master's licenses in four Samurai arts as well as a traditional healing art called Sotai-ho. Richard is one of the world's foremost experts in the traditional Japanese martial arts.

Through his books, his meditation and martial arts seminars, Richard Haight is helping to ignite a worldwide movement for personal transformation that is free of all constraints and open to anyone of any level. Richard Haight now lives and teaches in southern Oregon, U.S.A.

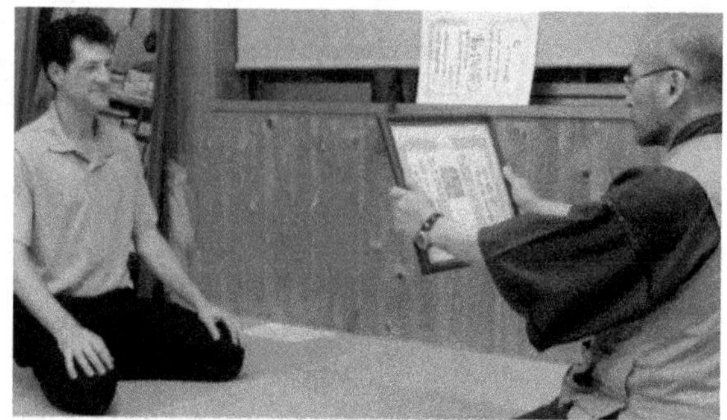

Receiving the License of Full Mastery from Master Shizen Osaki
Kanagawa, Japan, July 2012.

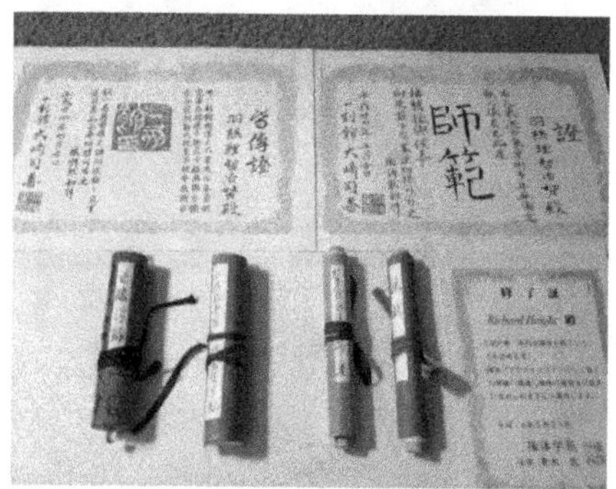

(Top—left to right) License of Full Mastery and Instructors License in Daito-ryu Aikijujutsu
(Mastership Scrolls—left to right) Daito-ryu Aikijujutsu, Yagyu Shinkage-ryu Hyoho,
Shinkage-ryu Jojutsu, Seigo-ryu Battojutsu, Sotai-ho (Master's License)

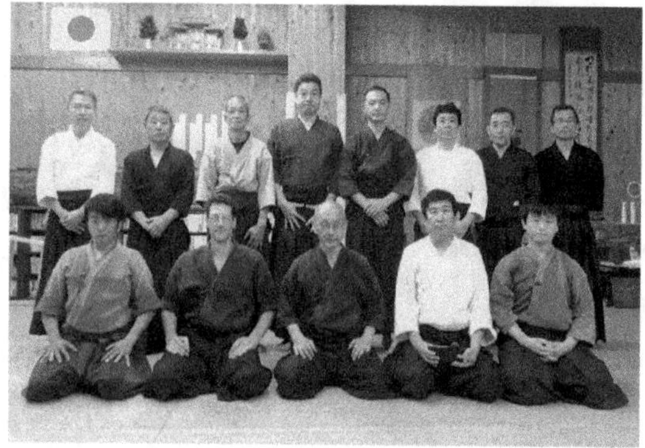

Front and Center, Shizen Osaki, Sensei
Kanagawa, Japan, October 2017

Sources

Bratic, Ana, and Nils-Görän Larsson. "The Role of Mitochondria in Aging." *Journal of Clinical Investigation* 123:3 (2013): 951-957.

"Hypothermia." Mayo Clinic. <https://www.mayoclinic.org/diseases-conditions/hypothermia/symptoms-causes/syc-20352682>

Pizzorno, Joseph. "Mitochondria-Fundamental to Life and Health." *Integrative Medicine* 13:2 (2014): 8-15.

"Raynaud's Phenomenon." Johns Hopkins Medicine <www.hopkinsmedicine.org/health/conditions-and-diseases/raynauds-phenomenon>

Spector, Dina. "The Odds of You Being Alive Are Incredibly Small." Business Insider 11 June 2012 <https://www.businessinsider.com/infographic-the-odds-of-being-alive-2012-6>

"Stunning Details of Brain Connections Revealed." ScienceDaily, 17 November 2010. <www.sciencedaily.com/releases/2010/11/101117121803.htm>

"Vagus Nerve." Encyclopaedia Britannica. Accessed 29 June 2020. <www.britannica.com/science/vagus-nerve>

Wigley, Fredrick M. and Nicholas A. Flavahan. "Raynaud's Phenomenon." *New England Journal of Medicine 375:6 (10 August 2016): 556–565.*

Contact

Here are some ways to connect with Richard Haight's teachings:

- Website: www.richardlhaight.com
- Publishing Notifications: www.richardlhaight.com/notifications
- YouTube: Tools of Spiritual Awakening with Richard L Haight
- Facebook: www.facebook.com/richardlhaightauthor
- Email: contact@richardlhaight.com

Step-by-Step Workbook

Chapter 1 – Neuroplasticity (page 11)

Am I stuck in my ways?

Yes No

What would someone who knows me well list as areas in which I am set in my ways?

-
-
-
-
-

What are my limiting beliefs?

-
-
-
-
-

What are some things I can do right now to help change those beliefs?

-
-
-
-

-

These are some stuck areas that I would like to change:

-

-

-

-

-

With the power of neuroplasticity, humans can intentionally strengthen any brain pattern. What are some healthy patterns that I want to reinforce today?

-

-

-

-

-

What did I do today to positively change my habits?

-

-

-

-

-

Rank your sleep quality over the next ten days by circling the description that best fits.

1. Poor Somewhat poor Okay Pretty good Like a Baby
2. Poor Somewhat poor Okay Pretty good Like a Baby
3. Poor Somewhat poor Okay Pretty good Like a Baby
4. Poor Somewhat poor Okay Pretty good Like a Baby
5. Poor Somewhat poor Okay Pretty good Like a Baby
6. Poor Somewhat poor Okay Pretty good Like a Baby
7. Poor Somewhat poor Okay Pretty good Like a Baby
8. Poor Somewhat poor Okay Pretty good Like a Baby
9. Poor Somewhat poor Okay Pretty good Like a Baby
10. Poor Somewhat poor Okay Pretty good Like a Baby

What are three things I can do to improve my sleep quality?

-
-
-

The sense of self changes with time. Here are some things about my sense of self that have changed over the years:

-
-
-
-
-

Plan a year's worth of positive emotional, thought, and behavior changes. These are the top five things that I will change over the span of a year:

-
-
-
-
-

Feeling uncomfortable is necessary to learn anything. In what ways did I intentionally challenge myself to move out of my comfort zone today?

-
-
-
-
-

Which negative or unhelpful habits do I most protect through denial or justification?

-
-
-
-
-

What are some of the mental dialogues that I use to protect negative habits?

____

____

____

____

____

____

____

____

____

In terms of priority, the negative habits that am most willing to let go of are as follows:

1.
2.
3.
4.
5.

Chapter 2 – Vagal Nerve Stimulation (page 18)

Did I practice vagal nerve stimulation today?

Yes No

How did I feel prior to vagal nerve stimulation?

Anxiety:

Extremely Low Low Average High Extremely High

Positive Motivation:

Extremely Low Low Average High Extremely High

Clarity:

Extremely Low Low Average High Extremely High

How did I feel after doing vagal nerve stimulation three times?

Anxiety:

Extremely Low Low Average High Extremely High

Positive Motivation:

Extremely Low Low Average High Extremely High

Clarity:

Extremely Low Low Average High Extremely High

Did I notice my pulse or blood-pressure change through vagal breathing?

Yes No Not Sure

What does it feel like doing vagal nerve stimulation three times?

____

____

____

____

____

____

____

____

____

Do I feel that practicing vagal nerve stimulation daily would be beneficial to my life?

Yes No Not Sure

Why do I feel this way?

____

____

____

____

____

____

____

____

____

Building on Chapter 1, how will I incorporate vagal breathing in my everyday life?

____

____

____

____

____

____

____

____

____

Chapter 3 – Other Bodily Changes (page 22)

From my own perspective, here is how I rank the strength of my blood vessels:

Very Weak   Weak   Average   Strong   Very Strong

From my own perspective, here is how I rank the strength of my mitochondria:

Very Weak   Weak   Average   Strong   Very Strong

Do I feel that having stronger blood vessels and healthier mitochondria will aid me to be more consistently awareness?

Yes   No   Unsure

Why do I feel this way?

____

____

____

____

____

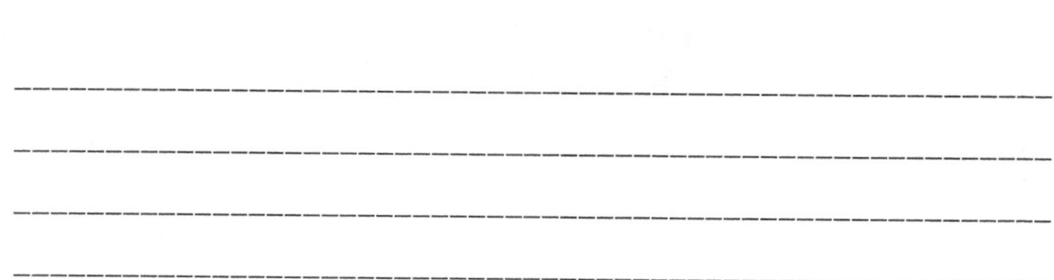

Does my answer come from extensive TEM experience, from something I was taught somewhere else, or from an assumption?

- Extensive TEM experience
- Something I was taught elsewhere
- Just my assumption

Chapter 4 - Primary Sounds (page 28)

Can I understand the perspective of the ancients with regard to sacred sounds?

Yes No Unsure

Can I feel the shift from beta brain wave to alpha brain wave while producing primary sounds?

Yes No Unsure

Did I notice that secondary sounds cannot be maintained throughout the breath as can primary sounds?

Yes No Unsure

Do I feel calmer and more aware after chanting primary sounds?

Yes No Unsure

Chapter 5 – Sound Dimensions (page 33)

Can I feel the "Ah" sound travel down my body?

Yes No Unsure

Once I have felt the dimensions of each sound, using one line for each, how would I describe the dimensions of each sound as I felt them?

Ah____

____

Ee____

____

Ew____

____

Eh____

____

Oh____

____

Mnn____

____

Nnn____

____

Chapter 6 – Sound Therapy (page 36)

Do I enjoy chanting primary sounds?

Yes No Unsure

How clearly am I currently able to find the sound and pitch which, to my body, feels most beneficial?

Not at all I get a vague sense I clearly feel the beneficial sound

How clearly am I currently able to find the sound and pitch to which my body feels most averse?

Not at all I get a vague sense I clearly feel the beneficial sound

Did I end the practice with the sound which is most beneficial?

Yes No Unsure

Chapter 7 – Purification by Water (page 41)

Absent the knowledge of science, can I relate to the ancient perspective of spirits?

Yes No Unsure

Can I see why the ancients thought cold water immersion exorcised evil spirits?

Yes No Unsure

What are some of the emotional experiences in my life that the ancients would describe as "spirits"?

____

____

____

____

____

____

____

____

____

What are some of the "spirits" in my partner, friends, or family members that I wish could be washed away?

____

____

____

____

____

____

____

What are some "spirits" in myself that I wish could be washed away?

Which negative emotions am I willing to wash away?

Chapter 8 - Facing the Water (page 44)

How did I feel just before starting the cold shower?

____

____

____

____

____

____

How did I feel just after the shower?

____

____

____

____

____

____

Did the practice change my emotional state and my energy level?

Yes No Unsure

Do I feel that Breath of Fire helped me to get control of my breathing?

Yes No Unsure

If Breath of Fire helped, about how long did it take to regulate my breathing?

About ___ second(s)/minute(s)

I was able to remain in the cold shower for ___ minutes.

Tomorrow, my aim is to remain in the cold shower for ___ minutes.

With safety and improvement in mind, which is the most appropriate approach to cold showers?

Full cold shower   Gradual Method   Sink Method

Has my approach to cold showers changed over time?

Yes   No

Chapter 9 - Flowing with Health Issues (page 53)

Do I experience symptoms of Raynaud's Syndrome? If yes, how should I care for myself, especially concerning cold showers and diet?

____

____

____

____

____

Do I have any other health issues that make taking cold showers especially challenging?

____

____

____

____

____

How does my health practitioner feel about my taking cold showers?

____

____

____

____

____

Chapter 10 - Measuring Progress (page 58)

Was I able to produce a steady, clear "Ah" sound while in the cold shower?

No Almost Perfectly

Were there any other primary sounds that I tried other than "Ah"? How did it go?

____

____

____

____

____

Have I noticed that my ability to produce primary sounds in the shower has improved with practice?

Yes No Unsure

How has my capacity to remain aware under stress changed as a result of practicing intentional cold showers?

____

____

____

____

____

Chapter 11 - Dealing with Dread (page 64)

Did I take a cold shower at the time of day when I was at peak energy?

Yes No Unsure

What was my degree of mental and physical resistance to taking the cold shower at peak energy? How long did I stay in the shower?

____

____

____

____

____

Did I take a cold shower when I was in a low energy state?

Yes No Unsure

What was my level of resistance to taking the shower in a low energy state? How long did I stay in the shower?

____

____

____

____

____

What was my inner dialogue about the cold showers?

____

____

____

____

____

Do I believe the thoughts and feelings of resistance are my true self, or do I feel that they are merely habitual neural pathways?

Yes No Unsure

Do I feel guilt or shame when I acknowledge those feelings and thoughts, or can I simply observe them?

Guilt Shame Both Guilt and Shame I simply observe them

Have I noticed the same resistant inner dialogues in other areas of my life outside of the cold shower experience?

Yes No Unsure

Here are the resistive dialogues that I experience during daily life.

-
-
-
-
-

What thoughts and feelings am I identifying as 'me' right now?

-
-
-
-
-

When and how do they come up during the day?

____

____

____

____

____

____

____

____

____

Have I noticed a lessening of identification with particular thoughts or feelings through cold shower pressure training?

Yes No Unsure

If you answered, "Yes", list the thoughts and feelings that have lessened their grip on your identity.

-

-

-

-

-

Chapter 12 Mentoring your Mind (page 70)

For the sake of mentoring my mind, do I use the gradual approach to the cold shower?

Every time Sometimes Never

Did the gradual approach help me to slowly build up to taking a full cold shower?

Yes No Unsure

Did giving myself choices lessen the resistance?

Yes No Unsure

Chapter 13 - Mentoring the Body (page 73)

Which avoidance strategies has my subconscious mind employed to avoid taking cold showers?

-

-

-

-

-

What percentage of the time am I able to successfully mentor my body into taking a cold shower?

Roughly _____%

Which negotiation strategies work most consistently for me? List them in order of effectiveness:

1.
2.
3.

Chapter 14 - The Power of One Breath (page 78)

Following the principle of one breath, what can I do to take immediate action on a goal, idea, or intention?

____

____

____

____

____

____

____

____

____

What ideas do I have that I can start on right now by writing them down?

____

____

____

____

____

____

____

____

____

____

Chapter 15 - Basic TEM Meditation (page 84)

Am I aware of when my mind is focused to exclusion?

Yes No Occasionally Unsure

Do I pay attention to the different states of mind during the day?

Yes No Occasionally

Do I get annoyed when something interrupts my focused concentration?

Every time Sometimes Rarely Never

During Visual Awareness Meditation, did I notice the difference between the alpha state of relaxed visual field and the beta state of focused attention?

Yes No Unsure

How do I feel before meditating as compared to during meditation?

____

____

____

____

____

____

____

____

____

How was my cold shower meditation experience? What were the difficulties? Was I able to remain meditated? What did I like about the experience?

____

____

____

____

____

____

____

Chapter 16 - Spherical Awareness (page 93)

How was my first spherical awareness meditation experience?

Was I able to experience spherical awareness in the shower during the first attempt?

Yes No Unsure

My first attempt at spherical awareness in the cold shower went like this:

____

____

____

____

____

____

____

____

____

Chapter 17 - Deeper Bodily Training (page 100)

What did I notice about taking a cold shower after charging my body with warmth?

____

____

____

____

____

Which is more challenging for my meditation right now, cold showers or cold baths?

Cold showers Cold baths Unsure

How was my first cold bath experience?

____

____

____

____

____

____

____

____

____

____

____

____

____

____

____

____

____

____

____

____

Chapter 18 - Awareness Exercises and Games (page 106)

Which exercises and games did I practice? Check mark them.

X-Ray Vision

Spinning with X-Ray Vision

Topographical View

Assassin Game

Notice Blind Spots

Gateway Awareness

Seat Positioning

Alternative Exits

Which are my favorite games and exercises? List the top three.

1.

2.

3.

What did I notice from playing those particular games and exercises?

____

____

____

____

____

____

____

____

____

Did I keep it light and fun?

Yes No Unsure

Are there any games or exercises that I don't like? List them.

-
-
-

Why don't I like those games and exercises?

____

____

____

____

____

____

____

____

____

____

____

____

____

Which exercises or games do I need to practice more? List them.

-

-

-

Chapter 19 - Daily Reminders (page 118)

I feel that time reminders are going to be helpful for me.

True False

I was successfully able to program my brain to remind me to meditate when I noticed the time.

True False

Which other types of reminders am using during my day?

-

-

-

-

-

-

Which type of reminder seems to work best for me? List them in order of benefit.

1.

2.

3.

Chapter 20 - The Heart of Chaos (page 124)

Have I ever noticed the voice of The Deceiver?

Yes   No   Unsure

I tend to notice immediately when the voice of The Deceiver comes up?

Never   Almost never   Occasionally   Often   Always

What was one of the dialogues of The Deceiver that I experienced today?

____

____

____

____

____

____

____

Where was it centered in my body?

Did I give in to the urges and compulsions of The Deceiver today? What was the urge or compulsion that I gave in to? What was the result?

If I was able to mentor my way out of following The Deceiver, how did it feel and what was the result?

____

____

____

____

____

____

Chapter 21 - Daily Embodiment (page 129)

I woke up sharp this morning.

Strongly agree Agree Unsure Disagree Strongly disagree

I give myself a powerful motivation to get up immediately upon waking up.

Strongly agree Agree Unsure Disagree Strongly disagree

I write my intentions for the next day the night before as a motivating force to get me out of bed in the morning.

True False

I practice primary sounds and take a cold shower upon arising.

True False

I play an awareness game to sharpen attention each day.

True False

I set reminders for myself in my environment to help me stay in spherical awareness throughout the day.

True False

Before going to bed, I take an accounting of the day by asking myself the following questions:

-

-

-

-

-

Did I notice 'The Deceiver' today? If so, was I able to soften the inner space and return to awareness?

Yes No Yes and No

Did I participate in any unhelpful habits and distractive comforts?

Yes No

What, if anything, did I do that was engaging but not meaningful?

____

____

____

____

____

Did I accomplish all the things that I aimed to do today?

Yes No

Did I set my aim to spend a bit more time in awareness than I did yesterday?

Yes No

Did I have fun with awareness?

Yes No

How did I get this day right?

____

____

____

____

____

____

____

____

____

____

____

____

____

____

Chapter 22 - Transformation (page 136)

What positive changes have I noticed that have come as a result of practicing the Total Embodiment Method?

It takes the average person about 66 days to establish a healthy habit, but it can take as much as a year for some individuals. A great way to help establish a healthy TEM practice it to keep a schedule of activities you will check off at the end of each day. Keeping up with this schedule every day will help you tremendously.

Please download the printable schedule.
www.richardlhaight.com/uaworkbook

Daily Guided Meditation Training with Richard Haight

If you would like more hands-on instruction about his meditation methods and teachings, you can get a 30-day trial of the TEM daily guided meditation service with Richard L Haight. Thousands of people are doing it every day!

Visit: www.richardlhaight.com/services

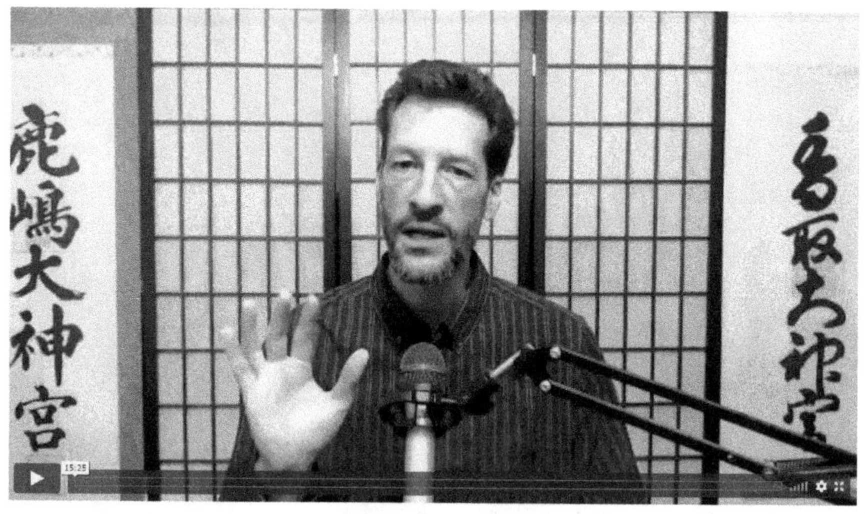

CPSIA information can be obtained
at www.ICGtesting.com
Printed in the USA
LVHW081027110920
665691LV00017B/1520

9 781734 965810